THE RELAXING ART OF

MASSAGE

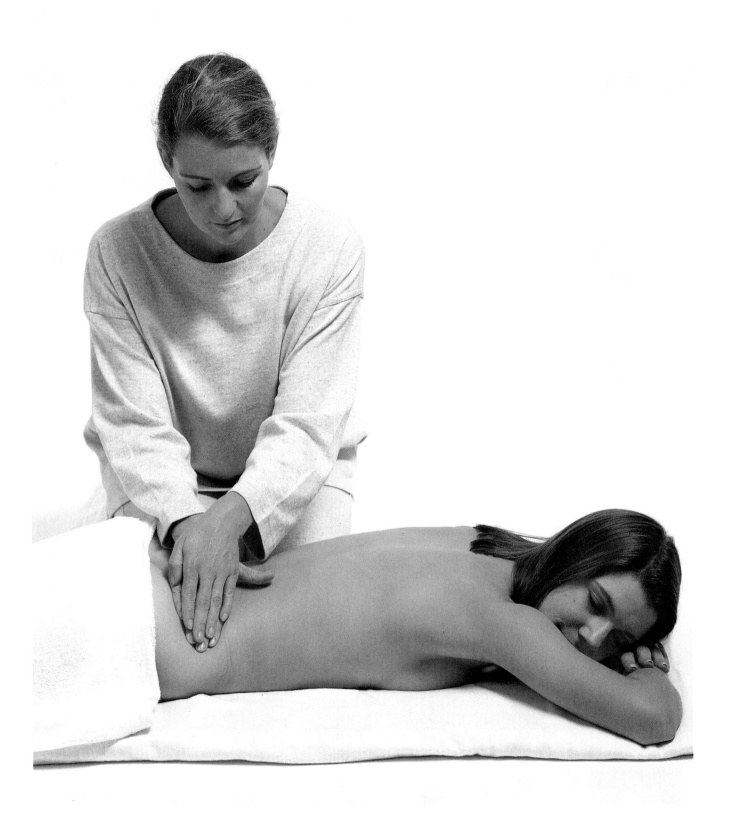

THE RELAXING ART OF
MASSAGE

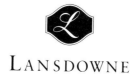

LANSDOWNE

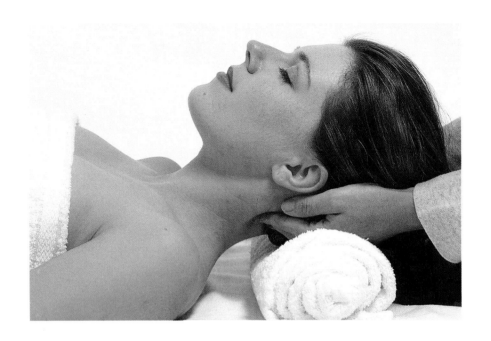

Contents

Chapter One

AN INTRODUCTION TO MASSAGE 6

Chapter Two

THE HISTORY OF MASSAGE 8

Chapter Three

APPROACHES TO MASSAGE 10

Chapter Four

PREPARATION 18

Chapter Five

BASIC TECHNIQUES 20

Chapter Six

THE FULL BODY MASSAGE 24

the back

the leg

the foot

the arm

the stomach

the chest

the neck

the face and scalp

Chapter Seven

A QUICK, DO-ANYWHERE MASSAGE 54

Chapter Eight

SELF MASSAGE 58

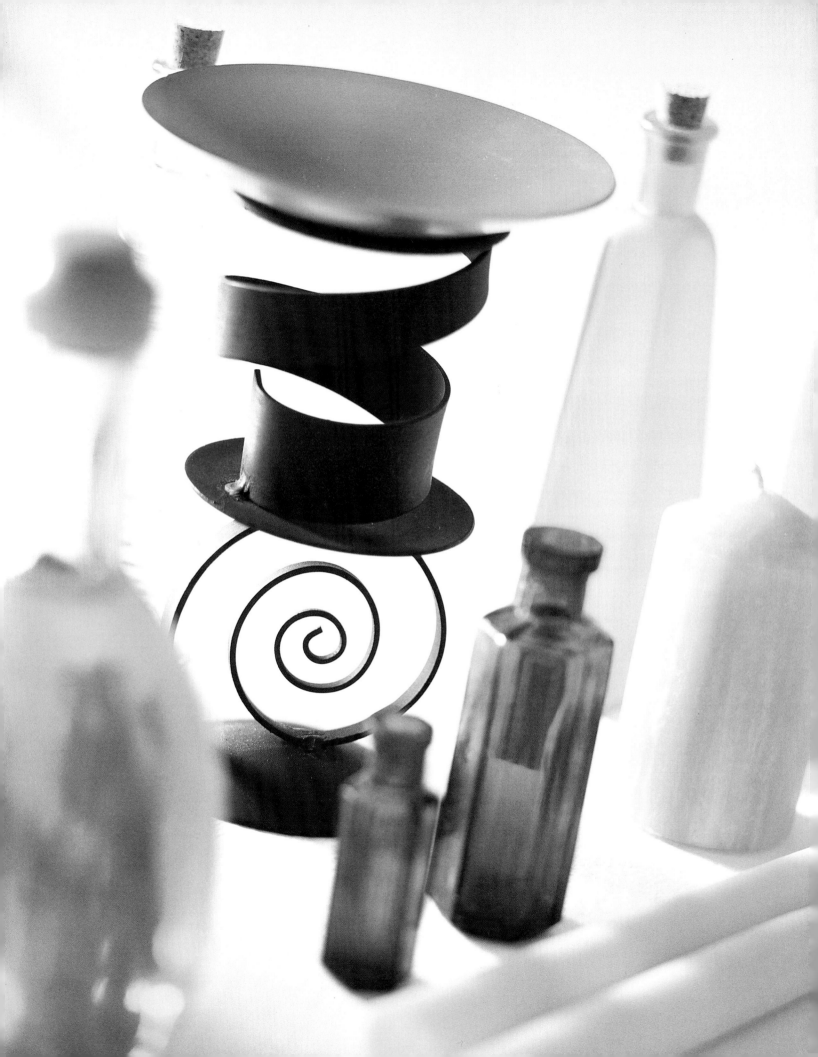

An Introduction to Massage

*O*f all the healing arts, massage is one of the oldest and the simplest. Everyday we unconsciously employ massage techniques because the desire and need to touch, and the action of touching, is instinctual. We stroke our temples to sooth a headache, we hold a friend's hand to comfort them, we "rub away" a child's knocks and bumps and if there is an injury we "kiss it better". Anyone can further develop this fundamental capacity for touch to provide physical and psychological benefits which are therapeutic to both the giver and the receiver of the massage.

In general terms, a massage is a systematic process of touch combining a number of techniques — such as stroking, friction, kneading, pinching, and pressing — in order to enhance health and wellbeing. There are a variety of massage therapies ranging from the traditional Swedish massage (which is often found in health spas, sports clubs, and gymnasiums) to acupressure, shiatsu, deep tissue, reflexology, and gentle aromatherapy massage. Massage is also used in conjunction with other therapies such as osteopathy and chiropractic.

The benefits of regular or even occasional massage therapy are extensive and often profound. The therapeutic and remedial physical benefits — when combined with the psychological benefits of conveyed warmth, understanding, and reassurance — can very quickly produce a secure, uplifted, even exalted sense of wellbeing.

Massage is a process of self discovery. In learning to massage, we learn to give and to empathize. In receiving a massage we learn trust; we learn how to accept such a gift. There is a feeling of communion, from which both people emerge with a new understanding of relaxation, peace, and vitality.

The benefits of massage

Most importantly, a massage makes us feel that someone cares about us, and this imparts warmth and happiness into our lives.

On a physical level, massage:
- relaxes the central nervous system
- soothes tight, tense, or overworked muscles
- removes toxins from the body
- improves circulation of blood and lymphatic fluid
- increases healing
- softens skin where scar tissue has formed
- breaks down fibrous tissue around joints
- prepares healthy muscle for demanding activity and aids recovery from this activity.

On an emotional level, massage can:
- calm the mind
- reduce stress
- relax or stimulate thought processes
- increase energy levels
- reduce apathy and depression
- soothe emotions.

The History of Massage

For thousands of years — probably since the existence of humankind — some form of massage or physical contact has been used to heal and sooth the sick, restore calm, and engender health and wellbeing. Massage is most likely the oldest form of medical treatment and evidence of its use can be found throughout history and across all cultures, from ancient times to the present.

Historical artefacts show that the Chinese were using massage techniques as early as 3000 years before the birth of Christ. The Ayurveda, Indian books written about 1800 BC, describe a process of rubbing and "shampooing" the body as a means of promoting recovery and healing of the body after injury. In both the art and literature of ancient Egypt, Persia, and Japan, many references are made to physicians employing the benefits of massage in an effort to counteract and heal many illnesses.

To ancient Greek and Roman physicians, massage was the first and principal method for treating and healing ailments and physical pain. Hippocrates, considered "the father of medicine", wrote in the fifth century BC: "The physician must be experienced in many things, but assuredly in rubbing...for rubbing can bind a joint that is loose and loosen a joint that is too rigid." Julius Caesar, an epileptic, was daily pinched all over to relieve recurring headaches and neuralgia, and Pliny, the renowned Roman naturalist, regularly received a "rub" to alleviate chronic asthma.

After the collapse of the Roman empire in the fifth century AD, massage fell in status and during the Middle Ages in Europe it came to be identified with the sinful pleasures of the flesh. The Renaissance of the sixteenth century, however, revived the therapeutic art. The work of two physicians — one a French doctor, Ambroise Pare, and the other an Italian, Mercurialis — became widely popular and fashionable, firmly re-establishing massage therapy as a legitimate and effective, albeit relatively elite, medical practice.

It was in the early nineteenth century, due to the developments by a Swedish practitioner, Per Henrick Ling, that massage took another leap forward and became commonly accessible and available. After travelling to the Orient as well as studying ancient Egyptian, Roman, and Greek techniques, Ling assembled a system of massage therapy known today as Swedish massage. In 1813 the first college to offer massage as part of the curriculum was established in Stockholm and in 1838 the Swedish Institute was opened in London. It is because of Ling's dedication and commitment that massage therapies are widely in use today.

Ling learnt the most about massage from studying Eastern methods because, unlike in the West, massage therapies have constantly held a highly respected position in these cultures and their use has continued in an unbroken line since prehistory. This positive attitude provided the perfect environment for experimentation which, over the centuries, has produced several different types of massage therapy.

Massage today is a dynamic practice which is constantly evolving, developing, and refining itself so there is a kaleidoscope of knowledge from which every individual can draw when developing their own style of massage.

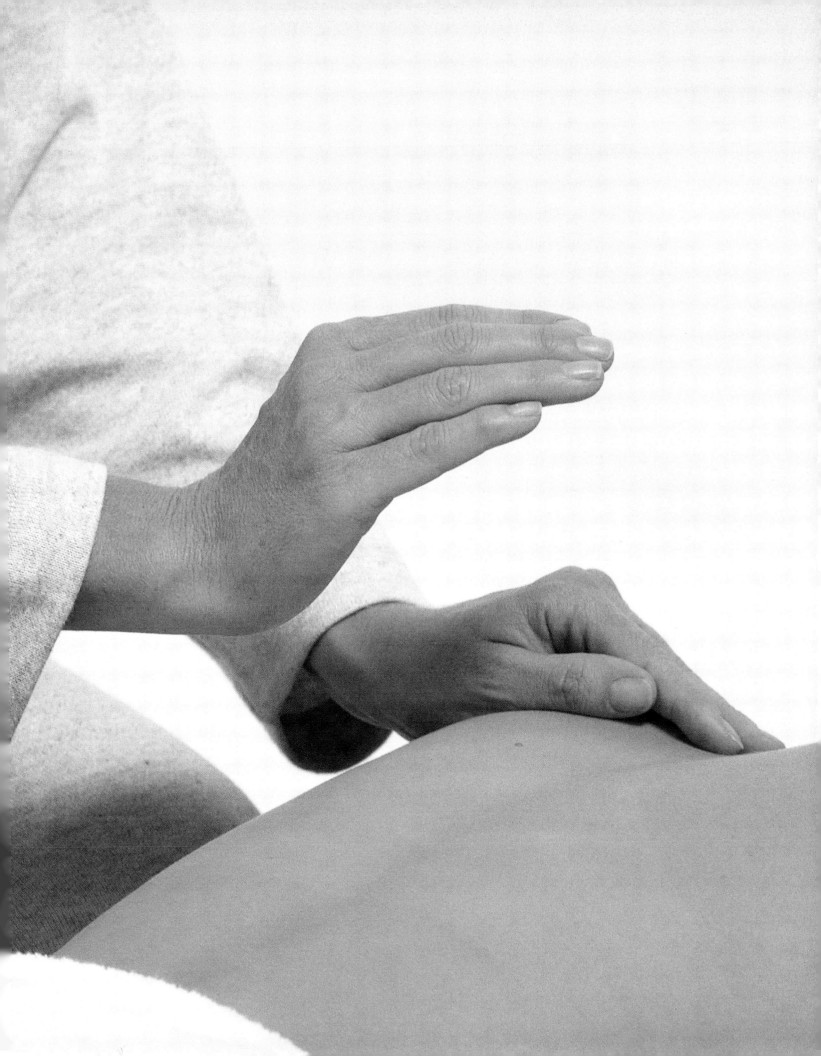

Approaches to Massage

The massage techniques you develop at home can be relaxed, spontaneous, and personal, but there is a huge variety of more formal massage styles from which you can learn and many kinds of practitioner whose help you can seek.

Massage is a two-way flow of touch and response, a mutual exchange. It involves the hands and the skin, which both give and receive — this is the medium for communication and the process through which healing energy can be experienced. These elements are common to all types of massage. However, when it comes to techniques and styles of massage, there is a vast array.

This chapter gives a brief description of some of the current styles of massage. There are many other massage techniques which you may wish to explore such as the rhythmic Hawaiian massage Lomi lomi, touch for health, and cranio-sacral therapy.

Of course, it is possible to incorporate several techniques into the one massage, for example a Swedish massage may be enhanced by use of acupressure.

Swedish massage

This is the most common form of massage in the Western world. It generally involves a full body massage with oils, and incorporates a number of basic massage techniques such as stroking, effleurage, frictions, petrissage, kneading, and percussion (see page 20). Depending on the techniques used, a Swedish massage may be relaxing or invigorating. The aim is to work on the soft tissues to soothe tight muscles and to stimulate the body systems.

Swedish massage is often accompanied by mood lighting, soothing music, aromas, and hot towels to enhance the atmosphere. This is an excellent style of massage to learn for use in the home and amongst friends.

Remedial massage therapies

Remedial massage uses more advanced techniques and may draw from several massage therapies. It is generally used to treat specific problem areas — for example, back and neck pain, shoulder pain, sprains, strains, respiratory problems, and sciatica. Like Swedish massage, it also stimulates the body systems. The process may involve a full body massage or concentrate on one or two areas. Techniques include soft tissue palpation, some deep tissue work, stretches, posture evaluation, therapeutic exercises, and pressure point therapy such as acupressure.

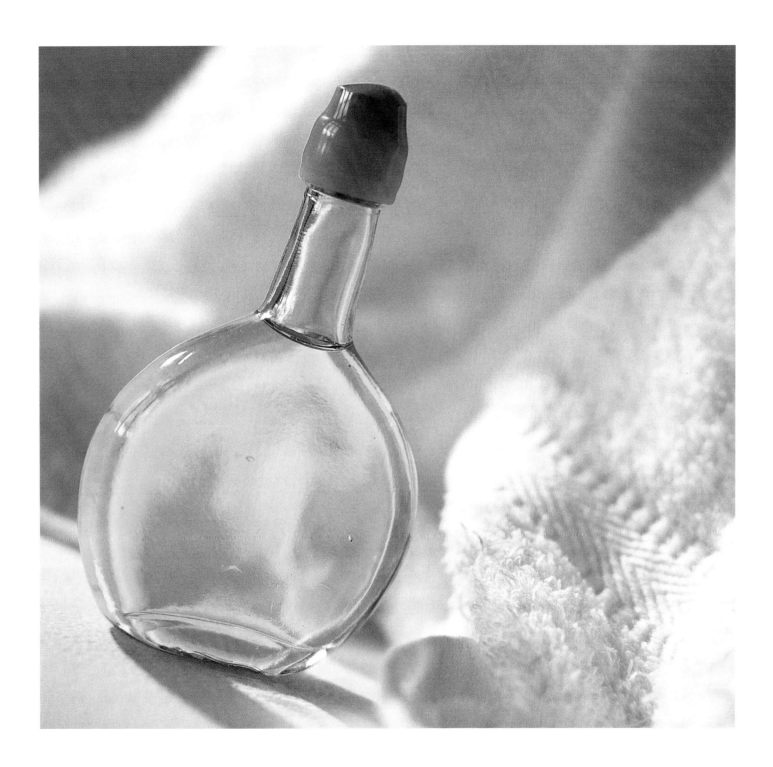

Deep tissue massage

After years of poor posture, stress, or misuse the body is often far removed from its "natural" postural state. Deep tissue massage helps reverse this process. Using pressure and gentle manipulation of the deep layers of soft tissue, it helps increase flexibility and reduce muscle tension and pain. The posture of the body is "resculpted".

As with all massage, emotional and psychological wellbeing is enhanced — it is thought that past trauma, physical and emotional, is stored deep within the muscular system. There are many styles of massage, such as Rolfing and Ka-Tone therapy, which make use of deep tissue techniques.

Sports massage

A form of remedial massage particularly suited to athletes. This massage method is used before physical exertion to tone muscles and joints which will help prevent injury and after exertion to treat any pain, muscle tightness, or injury.

Lymphatic drainage

The lymphatic system filters waste products and bacteria from the body, and plays an important part in fighting off disease. Massage can stimulate activity within this system. As the name suggests, the massage method known as lymphatic drainage is designed to flush the body of toxins and mucous. Techniques include deep muscular massage and the stimulation of lymphatic points, which become tender when the body is overloaded with toxins.

Positional release

A technique designed to alleviate and release painful muscle spasms in the body. The body has a number of surface "trigger points" which may suggest deeper muscular problems. The body is moved into various positions to reduce stress on the muscles, helping them to unwind and relax. This technique is very useful for headaches, muscle pain, poor posture, and fatigue.

Pressure point therapies

Acupressure

Put simply, acupressure is the application of pressure to acupuncture points instead of needles. Acupressure is based on the idea that there is an energy flow through the body which the Chinese call Chi or Qi. This energy circulates through the body along various pathways called meridians.

There are 14 main meridians in the body, each associated with a particular organ such as the heart, lung, gall bladder, and kidney. However, the function of the organ and its meridian is not necessarily interpreted in the same manner as in Western medicine. For example, if the liver meridian is not in balance, it will suggest problems in the area of blood storage and energy transformation, which will in turn result in emotional problems such as irritability and anger. It is often the case that the flow of Chi through a meridian can be blocked and stagnant, or adversely excessive. Such imbalances in energy flow will greatly impair health and vitality.

To counteract this problem, finger pressure is applied at specific points on the body. These points lie along the meridians and influence the flow of Chi within the meridian on which they sit. Usually, a finger or a thumb is applied to the point in a pressure-then-release, pressure-then-release action. Gradually the pressure will be increased until it is deep and constant. The pressure has to be exactly on the point for the treatment to work effectively. A point which is being worked will often feel tender.

The aim is to achieve a total balance within the body, and in this way health is achieved and maintained. Acupressure can easily be learnt and used at home as a self-help technique.

Tui Na

Tui Na is a form of Chinese massage based on the meridian system. It differs from acupressure in that a wide variety of hand movements are used to stimulate the points.

Jin Shin Do

This is a recent form of pressure point massage developed by an American woman, Iona Marsaa Teegurden. Jin Shin Do differs from acupressure in that it concentrates on releasing chronic stress in muscles. Called "armoring", this is tension that has developed over many years, often as a result of a stressful event, which is then gradually increased by other similar events that remind the person of the original trauma.

A gentle and prolonged form of pressure is applied, only increasing as the recipient relaxes and "invites" the deeper work. While the major point is being worked, several other points are also stimulated to enhance the release of tension and the return to balance.

Shiatsu

Shiatsu is the Japanese version of acupressure and, strictly translated, means "finger pressure". Other parts of the body, however — knees, elbows, knuckles, palms, and feet — are also employed in the technique.

The Japanese combined their traditional massage known as "anma" with the Chinese system of meridians. Rather like the Chinese, the lifeforce flowing through the meridian system is known as Ki. As in acupressure, it is imbalances in the flow of Ki which causes illness.

Shiatsu therapy diagnoses conditions by the state of the "hara" or abdomen, believed to be the area which indicates overall health. This diagnosis is of key importance to a successful treatment.

In shiatsu therapy the body weight is used to apply pressure to points along the meridians — there are over 600 points in total. Usually pressure is only applied for a short time. A variety of other techniques are also used as well as finger pressure; kneading, tapping, rubbing, and shaking, for example. Generally, the whole body is massaged in a number of "tonifying" sequences. The benefits are immediate, and symptoms fall away as the vitality (Ki) flows through the body.

Reflexology

Reflexology is strongly linked with the Chinese system of meridians. The idea is that the entire meridian system can be stimulated by working the feet and the hands because all of the meridians end or originate in either the hands or feet. Chinese medicine has always stressed that points located on extremities can have a powerful effect on the overall functioning of the body.

During the early 1900s, an American doctor, William Fitzgerald, became intrigued with this approach. He modified it slightly, called it Zone Therapy, and introduced it to the West. In Dr Fitzgerald's therapy, the body has 10 zones and the body's energy flows through these zones to reflex points in the hands and feet. Reflexology is based on the theory that by massaging points on the feet or hands, the related organ, body structure, or system (such as the lymph system) is stimulated, thus improving their performance and moving the body back to a state of health. Techniques include stroking, pressing, rubbing, and "walking" with the fingers and thumbs.

If you massage or "work" your own feet you may feel little crystals beneath the surface of the skin. It is believed that these are sediment deposits that settle in your body. Massaging can break up the deposits so they are absorbed and then eliminated. Care should be taken not to break up too many of these deposits during each treatment in case the waste elimination system is overloaded.

While massaging feet and hands, tender spots may also be located. This indicates that the energy relating to that area is out of balance.

Most reflexology treatments take between 45 minutes and an hour, covering the whole feet or hands. The main aim of reflexology is to increase the body's overall state of relaxation. As tension in the body is reduced, blood and energy supply improves throughout the body.

Reflexology can be learnt for home use and can be very beneficial as the feet are generally a much neglected area.

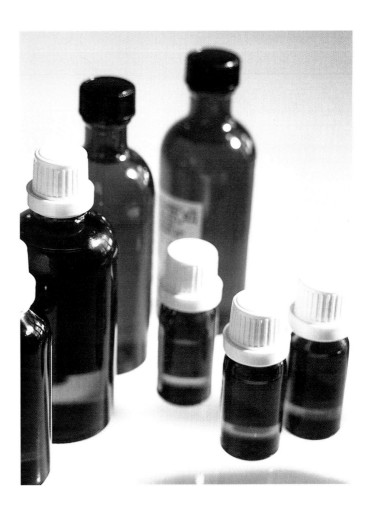

Aromatherapy massage

An aromatherapy massage combines massage techniques with the therapeutic use of essential oils. An essential oil is a highly concentrated extract from a plant substance — for example leaves, petals, bark, seeds, stalks, and flowers. The concentrate is very strong, capturing the living essence of the plant. Essential oils are readily absorbed by the skin and via the nasal passages, affecting both the physical and emotional planes.

Every essential oil has a different chemical composition, and thus a different influence on the body and mind. Depending on the oil chosen, an aromatherapy massage may be relaxing, invigorating, or uplifting (see the table on pages 14 to 17). Just add 10 to 25 drops of your chosen essential oil or oils to 2 oz (50 ml) of a neutral "base" or "carrier" oil, such as sweet almond oil.

Any massage technique can be used in conjunction with aromatherapy but the most common is the more gentle and relaxing form of Swedish massage. Aromatherapy can be easily adapted and learned for home use.

The Essential Oils

COMMON NAME	BOTANICAL NAME	PROPERTIES	CAUTION
Basil	Ocimum basilicum	Digestive • respiratory • soothing • calming • relaxing to muscles • head-clearing • uplifting • clarifying • aphrodisiac • mentally stimulating • aid to concentration • refreshing • useful for soothing skin abrasions	Avoid use during pregnancy.
Bay	Laurus nobilis	Soothing • relaxing • antibacterial • circulatory • anti-inflammatory	Avoid external use of bay if you have extremely sensitive skin, as it may provoke a rash.
Bergamot	Citrus bergamia	Respiratory • uplifting • clarifying • antiseptic • digestive • refreshing • useful treatment for skin and hair	This oil is phototoxic; do not use on the skin in sunlight.
Cedarwood	Juniper virginiana	Antiseptic • digestive • astringent • skin-toning • calming • aphrodisiac • harmonizing • strengthening • sedative • soothing	Avoid use during pregnancy.
Chamomile	Matricaria chamomilla (German), Anthemis nobilis (Roman)	Soothing • mildly antiseptic • analgesic • calming • relaxing to muscles • digestive • refreshing • balancing for the female system	Should not be used in the early months of pregnancy.
Clary sage	Salvia sclarea	Soothing • calming • relaxing • uplifting • euphoria-producing • warming • astringent • skin-toning • anti-inflammatory	Avoid use during pregnancy.
Clove	Carophyllus aromaticus	Antiseptic • antispasmodic • analgesic • nervine • carminative • digestive • respiratory • warming • slightly aphrodisiac	Avoid use during pregnancy.

COMMON NAME	BOTANICAL NAME	PROPERTIES	CAUTION
Cypress	Cupressus sempervirens	Balancing to the female system • stimulating • circulatory • respiratory • decongestive • head-clearing • antispasmodic • gently diuretic • refreshing • relaxing • astringent	Avoid the use of cypress oil if you suffer from high blood pressure.
Eucalytpus	Eucalyptus globulus	Anti-inflammatory • antispasmodic • analgesic • refreshing • stimulating • uplifting • cooling • invigorating • respiratory • head-clearing • decongestive • antiseptic • cleansing	Avoid if you suffer from high blood pressure or epilepsy.
Frankincense	Buswellia thurifera	Nervine • restorative • rejuvenating • comforting • relaxing • soothing • fear-dispelling • beneficial to the female system • respiratory	Avoid in the first three months of pregnancy.
Geranium	Pelargonium graveolens	Antiseptic • antidepressant • anti-inflammatory • diuretic • skin toning • refreshing • warming • relaxing • harmonizing • balancing	Avoid in the first three months of pregnancy.
Jasmine	Jasminum grandiflorum	Relaxing • uplifting • soothing • confidence-building • strong sensual stimulant • aphrodisiac • beneficial to the female system	Avoid use during pregnancy.
Juniper	Juniperus communis	Nervine • diuretic • analgesic • toning • cleansing • relaxing • balancing • refreshing • carminative • digestive • circulatory • appetite-stimulating • invigorating • relaxing to muscles	Avoid use during pregnancy.
Lavender	Lavandula officinalis	Head-clearing • respiratory • skin-healing • nervine • digestive • sedative • calming • balancing • refreshing • soothing • analgesic • antiseptic • antibacterial • decongestive • antidepressant • relaxing to muscles	
Lemon	Citrus limomum	Antiseptic • physically stimulating • skin tonic • astringent • antibacterial • diuretic • circulatory • refreshing • cooling • uplifting • stimulating • motivating	This oil can be phototoxic; avoid use on the skin in sunlight.

Choose an essential oil that suits your mood or your physical or emotional needs. You can use a combination of oils, but don't try more than three or four together.

COMMON NAME	BOTANICAL NAME	PROPERTIES	CAUTION
Marjoram	Origanum majorana	Antispasmodic • carminative • sedative • nervine • calming • relaxing to muscles • digestive • warming • fortifying • respiratory	Avoid use during pregnancy.
Myrrh	Commiphora myrrha	Digestive • respiratory • expectorant • anti-inflammatory • antifungal • astringent • antiseptic • tonic • stimulating • toning • strengthening • rejuvenating	Avoid use during pregnancy.
Neroli	Citrus aurantium	Antibacterial • healing to the skin • circulatory • digestive • nervine • calming • sedative • antidepressant • relaxing • fear-dispelling • aphrodisiac	
Orange	Citrus aurantium (bitter orange), Citrus sinensis (sweet orange)	Astringent • relaxing • refreshing • uplifting • antidepressant • digestive • antiseptic	
Patchouli	Pogostemon patchouli	Anti-inflammatory • nervine • sedative • relaxing • aphrodisiac	
Peppermint	Mentha piperita	Digestive • respiratory • anti-inflammatory • balancing to the female system • clearing • carminative • relaxing to muscles • refreshing • cooling (and warming)	
Pine	Pinus sylvestris	Respiratory • antiseptic • deodorizing • nervine • stimulating • refreshing • invigorating	Pine oil should not be used by people with sensitive skin, as it may cause skin irritation.

Essential oils should not be used directly on the skin.
Add 10 to 25 drops to about 2¹/₂ tablespoons of a neutral
"base" or "carrier" oil, such as sweet almond oil.

COMMON NAME	BOTANICAL NAME	PROPERTIES	CAUTION
Rose	Rosa damascena (rose otto), Rosa centifolia (rose absolute)	Antibacterial • antiseptic • astringent • anti-inflammatory • antidepressant • digestive • confidence-building • sensual • aphrodisiac • balancing • relaxing • soothing	Avoid in the first three months of pregnancy.
Rosemary	Rosemarinus officinalis	Digestive • nervine • respiratory • circulatory • muscular • invigorating • uplifting • stimulating • refreshing • clarifying	Avoid use during pregnancy.
Sage	Salvia officinalis	Diuretic • analgesic • antiseptic • decongestant • astringent • nervine • relaxing • refreshing • stimulating	Avoid use during pregnancy.
Sandalwood	Santalum album	Digestive • softening and healing to skin • antispasmodic • antidepressant • calming • relaxing • soothing • sedative • warming • confidence-building • grounding	
Tea tree	Melaleuca alternifolia	Antiseptic • antifungal • antibacterial • digestive • healing to skin • respiratory • decongestive • strengthening to the immune system	
Thyme	Thymus vulgaris	Antiseptic • disinfectant • circulatory • respiratory • nervine • stimulating • refreshing • fortifying • relaxing to muscles • strengthening to the immune system • cleansing and toning to skin	Avoid use during pregnancy.
Ylang ylang	Cananga odorata	Antiseptic • nervine • sedative • relaxing • soothing • balancing • antidepressant • aphrodisiac	

Preparation

*Whether it is a relaxing or an invigorating form of massage,
the aim is to calm, heal, and rejuvenate the body. The atmosphere and
tools, therefore, are important to the general effect and success.*

Creating the environment

Privacy

It is important for both you and your partner to be able to
switch off and escape from everyday noises for best effect.
Disconnect the telephone or switch on the answering
machine. Place a "do not disturb" sign on the door. Close
any windows or doors that let in outside sounds.

Music

Soft music played in the background will encourage
relaxation and promote concentration. Do not play music
too loud or it will defeat its purpose. An alternative to
music is a recording of natural sounds such as the sea or
birds. Such recordings lull the mind and help transport
your partner away from the scene of daily stress.

Lighting

Subtle lighting is very important. Bright, glaring lights
make it difficult to relax. Candlelight is ideal. It is useful to
have an eye patch handy to place over your partner's eyes
when lying on the back.

Room temperature

The room should be comfortably warm, but not hot. Drafts
should be eliminated. During summer a small fan can be
directed at you, but not your partner, as body temperature
drops during a massage.

Fragrance

A vaporizer, lightbulb ring, or burner using one of the
relaxing essential oils can be beneficial. Alternatively a
stick of incense can be burnt. Remember that the
fragrance must be pleasant to both people and scenting the
room is not necessary for aromatherapy massages.

Accessories

The best place to massage at home is on the floor (unless
you have a professional massage table). The person
receiving the massage can be supported by a thin foam mat
or folded blankets covered by a sheet or towel. This should
provide enough cushioning and comfort without being too
soft. A thick soft mattress or futon is NOT recommended
as it will counteract much of the pressure you apply. You
will also need to have on hand two pillows, several towels
(bath and hand size), an extra blanket or towel, and
possibly a hot water bottle for the feet.

Massage oils

You can use a commercial massage oil, or simply use an oil
from the kitchen — olive, sunflower, safflower, and coconut
oils are all suitable. Almond, avocado, and walnut oils can
be used but are very rich — they are best in winter months
or to enhance other oils. Cold pressed oils are preferable.
You can add few drops of an essential oil to the base carrier
oil. Keep the oil in a handy position throughout the
massage. Store in a dark glass container in a cool dark place
between uses. Watch that your oils don't turn rancid —
a small amount of Vitamin E or wheatgerm oil added to the
massage oil can prevent oxidization and thus lengthen your
oil's life.

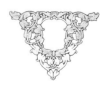

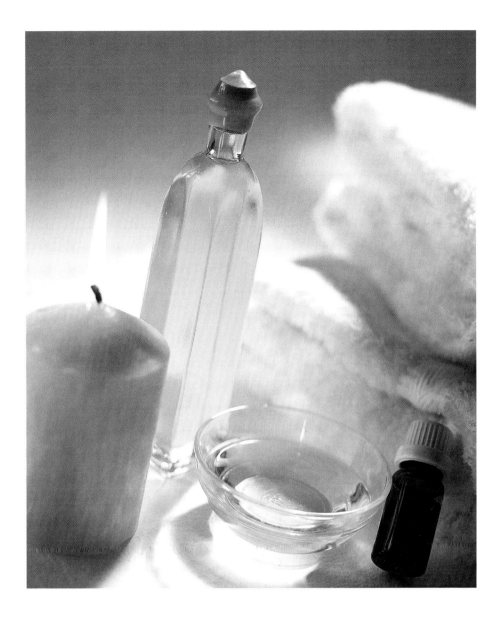

Giving a massage

Massage is a two way experience to be enjoyed by both participants. It is of vital importance that you are relaxed, calm, and comfortable throughout the treatment. Any tension, discomfort, or annoyance will be communicated to your partner and counteract any therapeutic benefit. Make sure that the atmosphere you have created for your partner is pleasant for you as well. Wear loose clothing; tight clothes and shoes will restrict your movement and even your circulation. Clean hands are essential. Thoroughly wash hands and scrub nails; long nails may need trimming. Clean and refreshed hands also allow for greater sensitivity. Exercise your hands regularly and particularly as a "warm up" before beginning a massage.

This will increase sensitivity and flexibility and reduce the possibility of strain from applying pressure. A few simple exercises to try are:
• Squeeze and release a small rubber ball with one hand. Repeat about a dozen times with each hand.
• Holding the tip of a finger with the thumb and forefinger of your other hand, gently rotate the finger in one direction, then the other, then gently pull away from joint. Repeat for all fingers on each hand.
• Place your hands together. Keep your fingers together but move your elbows out so that your palms no longer touch. Press your fingers together firmly and hold for a few seconds. Repeat a few times.

The Basic Massage Movements

*In Swedish massage, there are a number
of basic techniques which are very useful to learn, as they are
frequently repeated throughout the massage.*

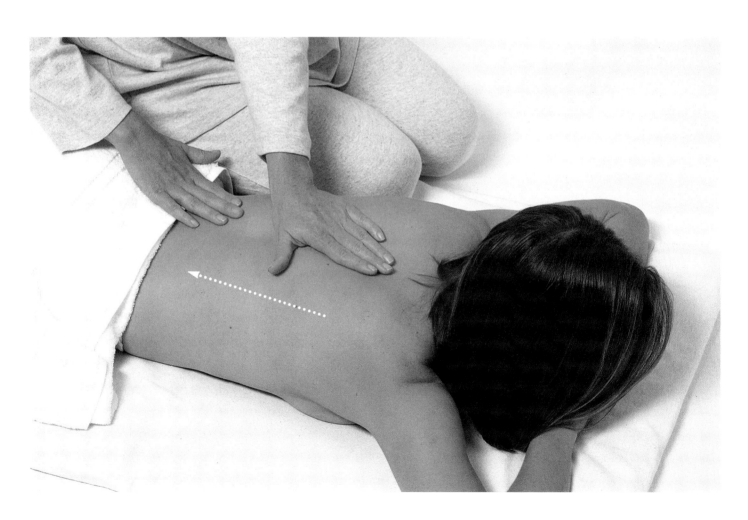

Stroking

Stroking is very important as it establishes the first contact with your partner and helps you to locate areas of muscle tightness or pain. Use long, gentle strokes to spread oil over the area being massaged. Stroke with both hands at once, or alternate. On the legs or arms, stroking is usually in the direction of the feet or hands. Stroking should always be relaxing, soothing, and comforting — use a light touch.

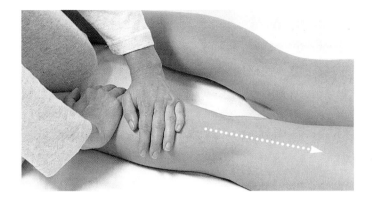

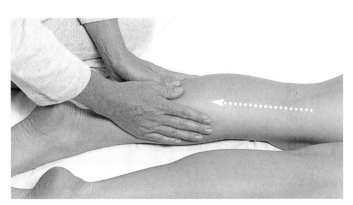

Effleurage

Effleurage warms the area being massaged and promotes circulation. It also has a relaxing effect on tight, tense muscles.

Effleurage is generally a long, even stroke applied with firm pressure. It is a movement that has two parts.

First, slide your hands forward. Generally, both hands work at the same time, either side by side with thumbs touching, or one below the other as illustrated in the first picture. When used on the back of your partner, you may move your hands in any direction, but on the limbs the movement should always be in the direction of the heart — this is the opposite to stroking.

Second, after sliding hands forward, draw them back lightly in the opposite direction, as in the second picture.

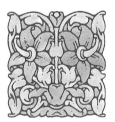

Petrissage

Petrissage helps to relieve muscle fatigue and eliminate the buildup of toxins. It includes a range of movements, such as kneading, rolling, wringing and squeezing. While stroking and effleurage are long, gliding movements, petrissage concentrates more on specific muscle areas to "soften them up" for deeper massage.

Kneading in a massage is just like kneading bread. Use each hand alternately to hold and squeeze flesh between your fingers.

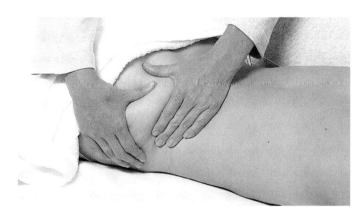

Frictions

Frictions work at a deeper level, concentrating on just a small section of the body at one time. This movement is designed to penetrate problem areas of tension buildup.

Generally the pads of your thumbs or fingers are used to create small circular movements. It is also possible to use the heel of your hand. Work slowly and carefully into the area — start gently and increase pressure as you feel the muscle tissue relaxing beneath your fingers.

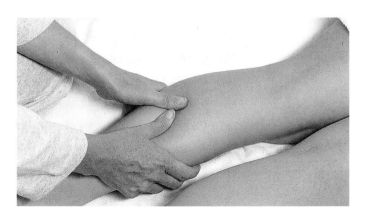

The technique shown on these two pages is known as percussion. If the aim of the massage is to quietly soothe your partner, percussion may be too vigorous. However, it can be a great stress reducer and very uplifting.

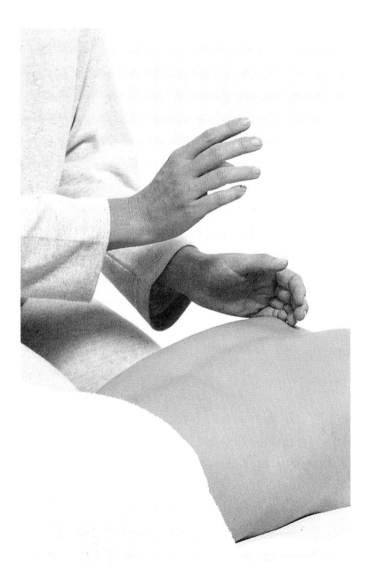

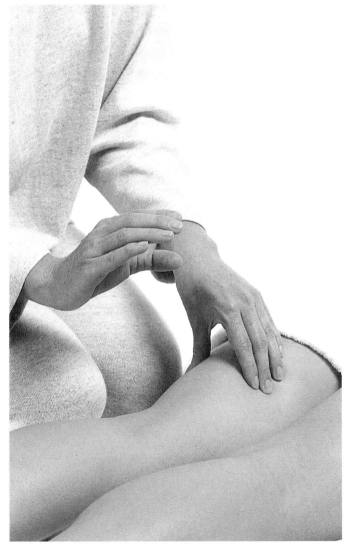

Flicking

Also known as hacking. In this movement the hands are relaxed, with palms facing one another. Use the little finger side of your hands and gently flick the surface of the skin with one hand and then the other. Keep your hands close together and try to form an even rhythm. The hands should be loose, bouncing easily off your partner's skin.

Plucking

This is a gentle and fairly rapid movement. Pick up the flesh between your thumb and fingers and then release, creating a plucking movement. Alternate the plucking from hand to hand to form a smooth rhythm.

If you do decide to use percussion movements,
follow with flowing movements such as stroking.
Make sure to keep your wrists loose,
and use only light percussion on bony areas of the body.

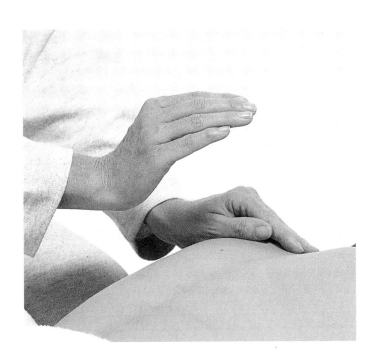

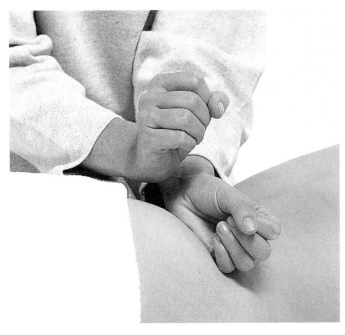

Cupping

Once again, keep wrists loose but form the hands into a cupped position, fingers touching lightly. The hands should be arched at the knuckles, forming a cavity. Each hand cups the surface of the skin alternately, keeping an even beat. This movement should create a loud, hollow sound.

Pounding

Also known as pummelling, in this movement the hand is held in a loose fist. Use the little finger side of the fist, one hand after the other, to gently pound the muscle mass. Lift your fist off the skin straight away, creating a light, springy motion.

CAUTION

Percussion movements are generally done on healthy persons. Do not use if your partner has:

— any bone fractures

— experienced spasms or exaggerated reflexes

— very little body fat

— a very reactive or nervous nature.

Do not use at all behind the knee, over the kidney area, or along the spine.

Vibrations

Vibrating movements can help to create warmth, to soothe stiff joints and muscles, and aid chest conditions. Vibrations can be soothing or invigorating. If the desire is to soothe, use the flat of the hand and allow energy to pass from you to your partner in a vibrating motion. For a deeper, more invigorating effect, try creating vibrations with the end of your fingertips. These movements are difficult to describe or illustrate, but with practice you will be able to confidently generate this vibrating sensation.

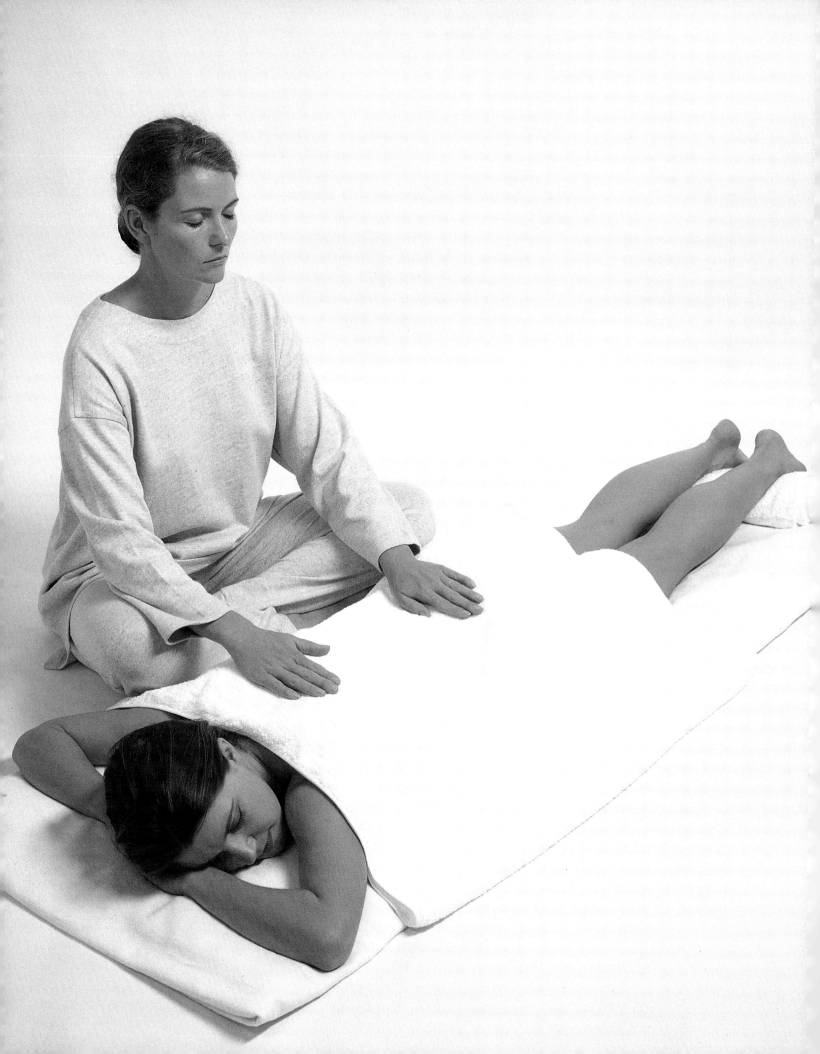

A Full-Body Massage

The most important parts of a massage are
the beginning and the end. The initial touch will set
the mood of the massage for both of you.

Try to maintain contact with your partner's body at all times during the massage; even when moving into a new position, try to keep one hand on the body.

• When massaging different parts of the body, keep the rest of the body covered with a large towel or blanket. This will keep your partner warm — this warmth will not only be soothing but shall also assist the therapeutic benefits of the massage and increase the absorption of oils used.

• Try not to talk too much throughout the massage as it will interrupt the process but do encourage your partner to let you know if there is any discomfort or a particular need.

• Always ensure your hands are warm before placing them anywhere near your partner — rub briskly together if they are at all cold.

A full body massage can be performed in any order. It is common to begin with the back or back of the legs, progressing to the front of legs, arms, abdomen, chest, and finishing with the neck and face.

Connecting

Once your partner is comfortable and covered by a blanket or towel, gently place your hands on their body — one hand on the nape of the neck and the other on the small of the back, for example. Breathe slowly and deeply, close your eyes and let the energy flow between you. Very softly rock your partner's body from side to side. Focus in this position for several minutes before allowing your hands to lift from the body. Now you are ready to fold back the covering and begin massaging.

Watch your posture or you'll end up sore and tired. Keep your back as straight as possible, your shoulders relaxed, and your head balanced above your spine. If you are not comfortable in any position, move to one where you are. Remember to use the weight of your body when applying any pressure to lessen strain on yourself.

The Back

Your partner should be lying face down with the head turned to one side — changing the direction of the head occasionally will prevent a stiff neck. Position the arms where they are comfortable and a pillow under the ankles for support.

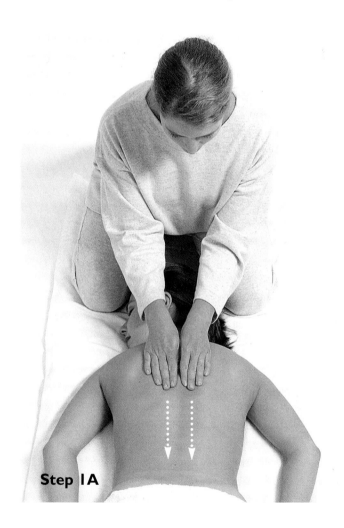

Step 1A

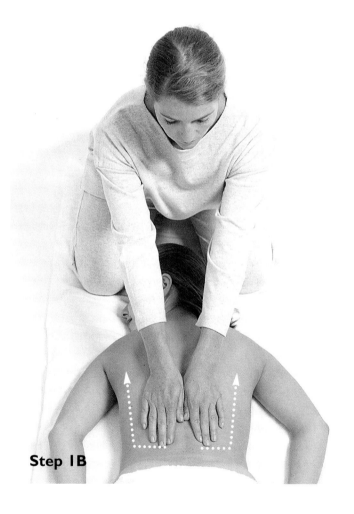

Step 1B

1. Kneel near the head of your partner and apply a light coating of oil with long gentle stroking movements over the entire back and shoulders.

Using effleurage strokes, glide your hands down each side of the spine then slide them back up the side of the body. It is best to have your hands side by side with thumbs close together. Let your body lean into the movement as you work down the body and draw back as you move your hands back towards the shoulders.

Repeat several times.

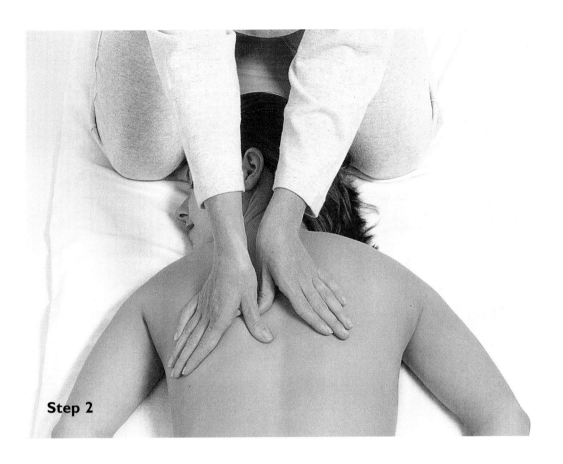

Step 2

2. Work the muscle which runs each side of the spine.

Using friction movements, move your thumbs in circles from the top of the spine to the base — then return up the sides of body in a sweeping movement.

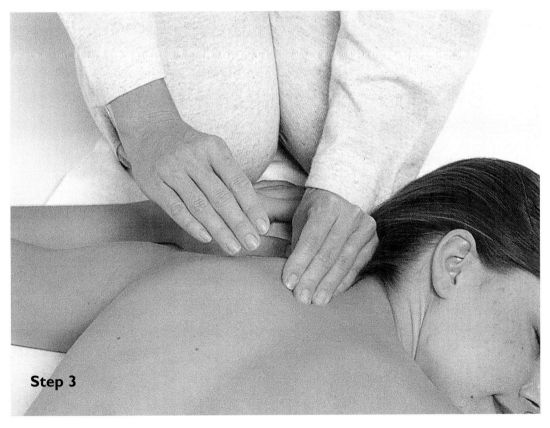

Step 3

3. Moving on to the shoulders, knead the upper shoulder muscles. Gently squeeze and release around the whole shoulder area.

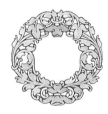

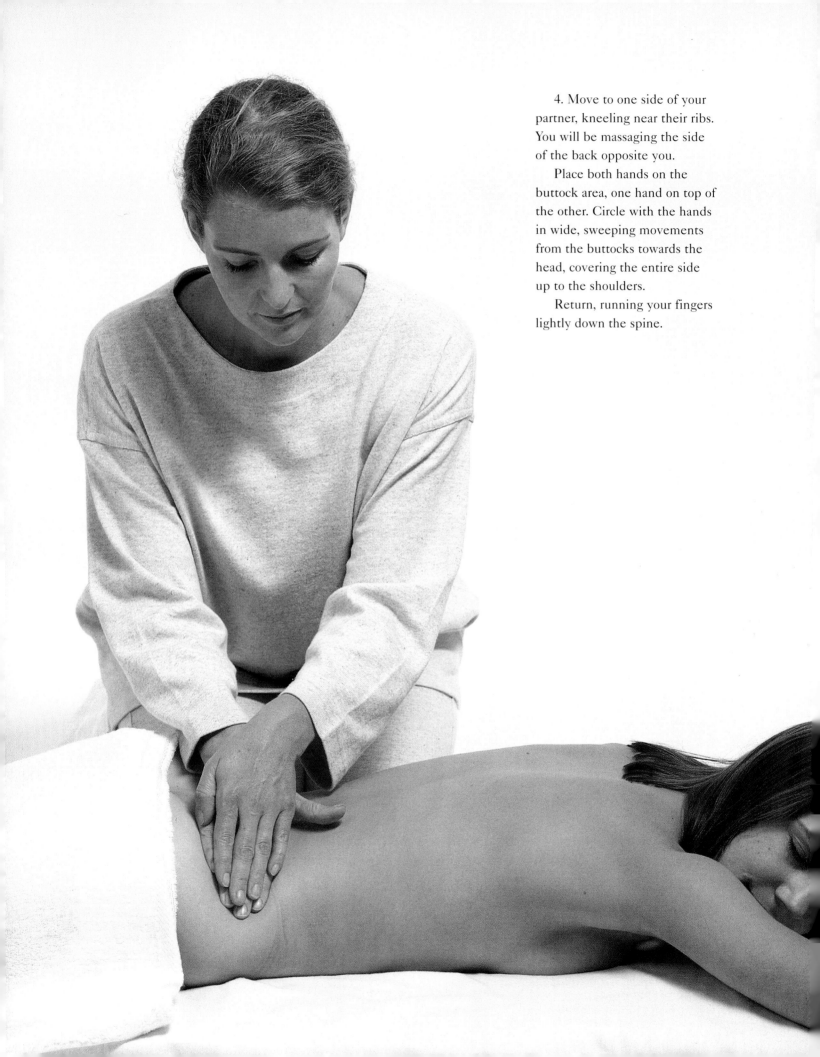

4. Move to one side of your partner, kneeling near their ribs. You will be massaging the side of the back opposite you.

Place both hands on the buttock area, one hand on top of the other. Circle with the hands in wide, sweeping movements from the buttocks towards the head, covering the entire side up to the shoulders.

Return, running your fingers lightly down the spine.

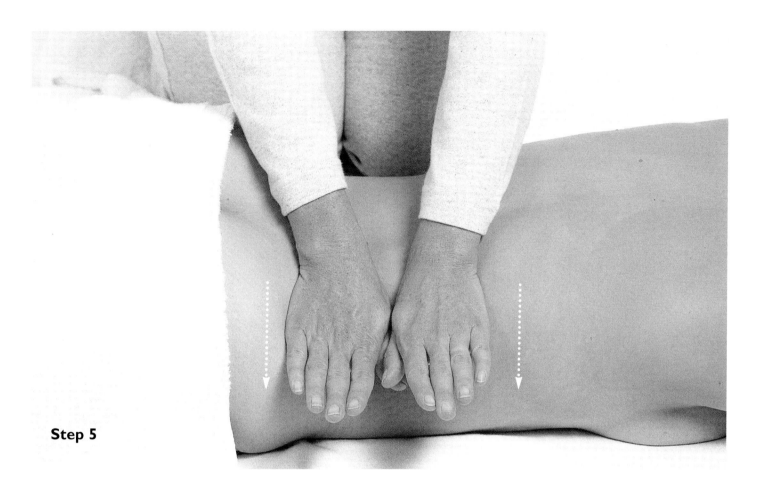

Step 5

5. On the same side of the body, knead the flesh with the heels of your hands.

Start at the buttocks with your hands side by side, and push away from the spine with the heels of both hands.

Pull back lightly with your fingers, feeling the flesh roll beneath. Work all the way to the shoulders and back to the buttocks with this movement.

After completing
step seven, move to the other side
of your partner and repeat
steps four to seven.

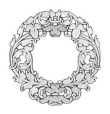

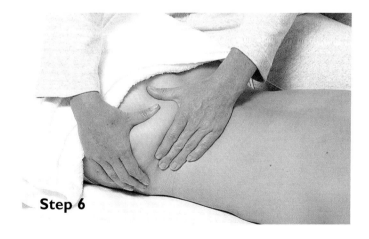

Step 6

6. Knead the buttock area on the side opposite you, using squeezing and releasing movements. Many people store tension in their buttocks — knead it away.

7. Work a little deeper with frictions over the buttock and base of spine. Use the pads of fingers to locate and work tight muscle areas. Do not press too firmly on the bones at the base of the spine.

8. Kneel near the shoulder of your partner. It may be easiest if you lift your partner's arm and place their forearm on their lower back as shown.

Slide your hand under their shoulder for support. Use your fingertips and the circular friction movement to massage the shoulder blade.

Stroke along the edge of the shoulder blade using the side of your finger.

Try to raise the shoulder blade by lifting the shoulder with your other hand — now you should be able to reach underneath the bone to the muscle.

Change sides and repeat.

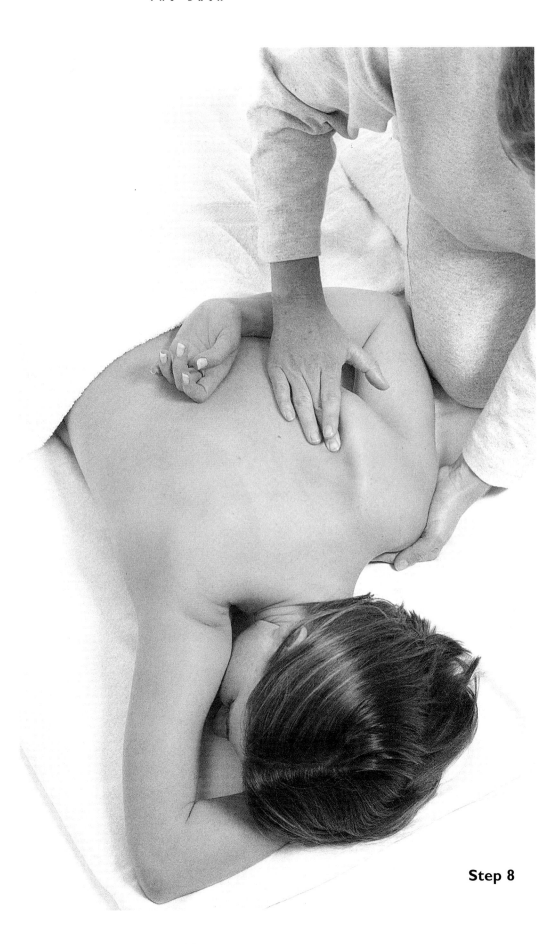

Step 8

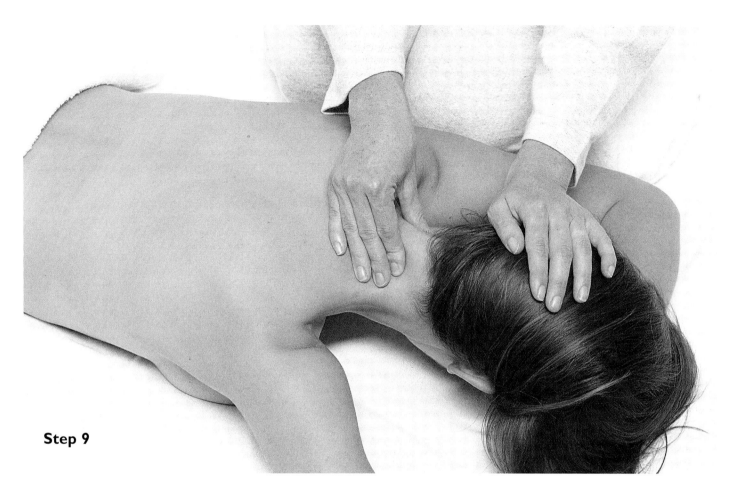

Step 9

9. Now knead the neck with your thumbs and fingers. Pick and squeeze the flesh, working the area thoroughly. The neck will be massaged fully later in the massage.

10. Move to sit beside your partner's lower back. Effleurage lightly, from the base of the spine to the shoulders, gliding up the middle of the body with your hands on each side of the spine, and continuing in a smooth movement across the shoulders, returning down the sides.

If desired, percussion movements and vibrations can be used to warm the area before the effleurage (see page 22 and 23). Remember to avoid the kidney area, all bony protusions, and the spine.

To finish the back, move to the head of your partner, and gently stroke from base of spine to neck. Cover the back with a towel and pat gently.

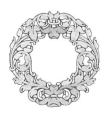

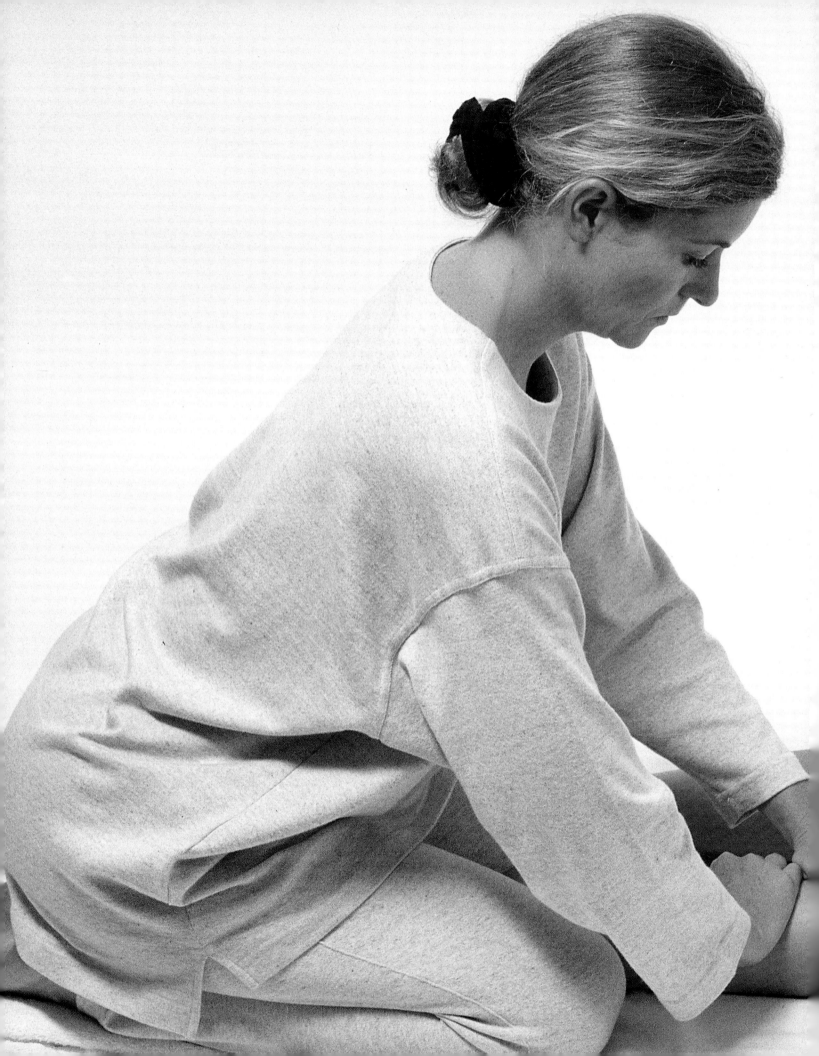

The Leg

*It is recommended that you uncover
one leg at a time, keeping the remainder of the body
covered and warm. You could also try placing
a pillow under the shin as it relieves pressure
from the lower back.
Kneeling near the foot of your partner,
apply oil with gentle stroking
movements covering the entire leg,
from thigh to ankle, then follow with effleurage.*

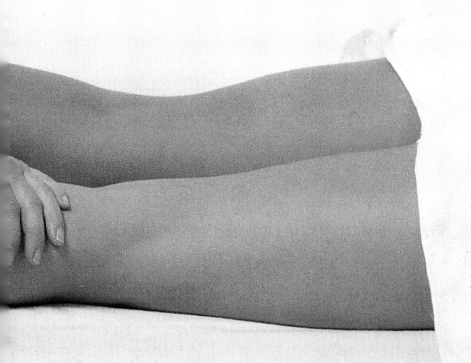

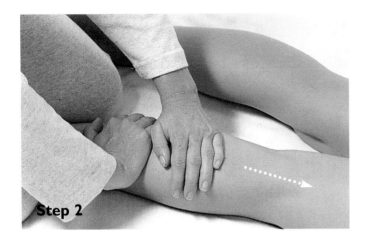

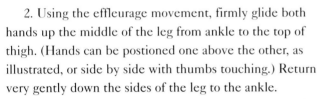

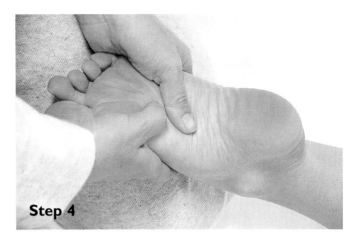

2. Using the effleurage movement, firmly glide both hands up the middle of the leg from ankle to the top of thigh. (Hands can be postioned one above the other, as illustrated, or side by side with thumbs touching.) Return very gently down the sides of the leg to the ankle.

The movement should be firm on the upwards motion and gentle on the downwards. Remember to keep your back straight and move your body with the movement.

3. Kneel or sit cross-legged near your partner's toes and cradle the foot in one hand, lifting it off the ground. Stroke the foot firmly with the other hand.

4. Rest the foot on your knee or in your lap and use your thumb in the friction movement to massage in small circles over the entire sole. Alternate between the thumbs. The feet will be massaged more fully later in the massage (see page 36).

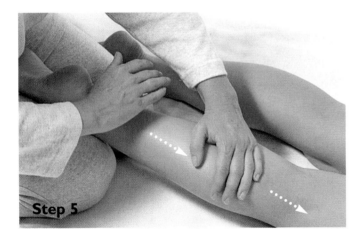

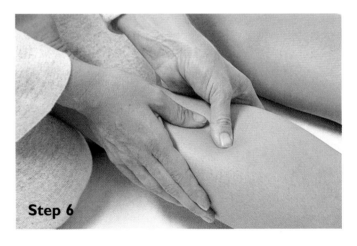

5. Now work on the calf of the leg — you may find it comfortable to place your partner's leg on your knee.

The movement is a firm effleurage stroke, using only one hand at a time. Cupping your hands, stroke up the calf muscle with one hand — as it reaches the top of the calf, the other hand begins with the same movement from the ankle to form a rhythmic, flowing motion which is very warming to the muscle.

6. Having relaxed the area, now work more deeply into the muscle mass using circular thumb frictions.

It is best to work up the calf, circling upwards and outwards with the thumbs. Begin gently, increasing pressure gradually — many people are very sensitive in this area.

7. Next, move up to the thigh, repeating the same effleurage and friction movements.

Thoroughly massage the back of each leg in turn.
Your partner should then roll over so that you can work gently
on the front of the legs.

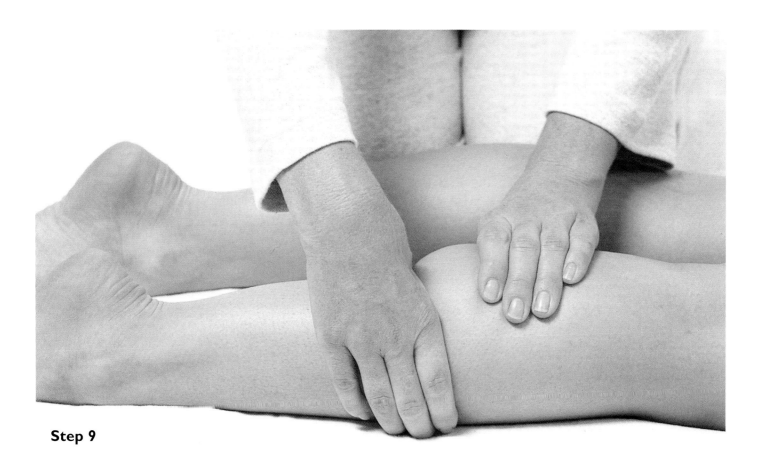

Step 9

8. Reposition yourself beside your partner's knee as the following movements are worked on the whole leg. Knead the flesh from thigh to ankle, then back up to the thigh.

9. Introduce a wringing movement, starting at the calf and working up the leg to the thigh. The hands are held side by side, as illustrated above, one pushing as the other is pulling. Use a firm pressure but be careful not to pinch your partner.

10. You may like to try a series of percussion movements (see page 22 to 23) if appropriate. Such movements feel very stimulating on the back of the legs and pounding can be used on the large thigh muscle. Avoid the area around the back of the knee when using percussion movements. Start very gently.

11. Finish with effleurage to the entire leg.

12. End by softly drawing your fingers over the foot and off the edge of the toes.

13. Cover leg with a towel and pat gently.

14. Repeat entire process on the back of the other leg.

15. *Ask your partner to roll over onto their back.* Cover again with towels and place a pillow under the knees for support. You may like to place a thin pillow under the head and a patch or cloth over the eyes to block out the light.

16. Repeat the same process on the front of the legs but concentrate on the upper thigh. Remember there is no real muscle mass on the front of the lower legs so stroking and gentle kneading is all that is required. Avoid the bone area as this is very sensitive.

Massage the front of one leg at a time, and don't forget the feet (see page 36).

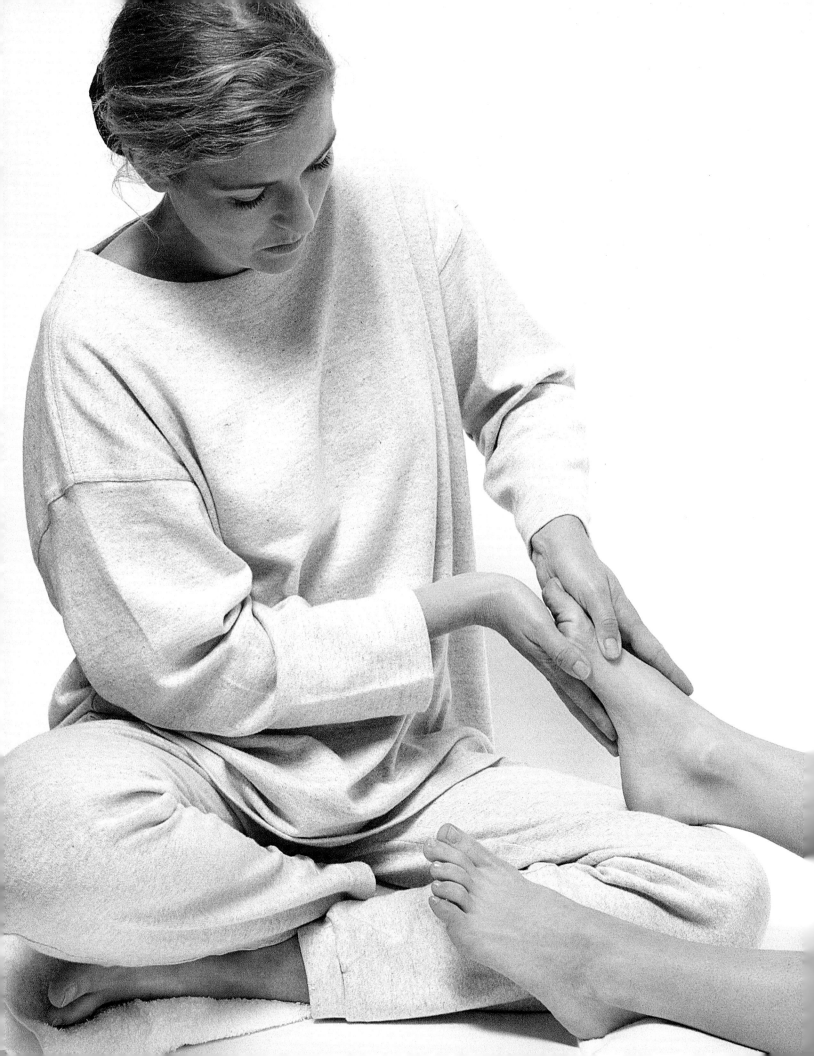

The Foot

Receiving a foot massage while lying on the back tends to be more relaxing for most people. Remember to begin with firm pressure as people can be ticklish in this area.

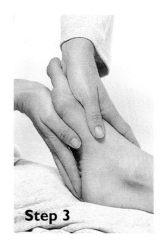

Step 3

3. Cup the foot with both hands, thumbs towards the midline of the body, and effleurage the whole foot with firm stroking movements. Your hands should travel the whole length of the foot.

4. Move down to the ankles, circling the ankle bones with the pads of the fingers — cover the area around and behind the ankles.

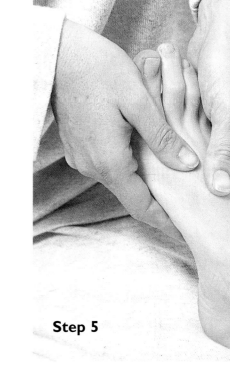

Step 5

A full foot massage should be incorporated into the leg massage. After massaging the front of one leg, shift your attention to the foot. Then repeat the whole process on the other leg — massage the front of the right leg then the right foot, for example, then the left leg and the left foot. Do not keep switching from leg to leg.

If the temperature is cool, you can cover the rest of the leg while concentrating on the foot.

1. Kneel or sit cross-legged at your partner's feet. You may like to place the foot on your knee or in your lap. This can be tricky so you may want to experiment with different postions.

2. Rub your hands together briskly to ensure they are warm, then apply oil to the foot in a stroking movement.

5. Work the top of the foot. Support the foot with your hands as illustrated, and stroke the top of the foot with your thumbs. Glide thumbs between the small bones of the feet, feeling for the furrows between the bones.

6. Sandwich the foot between the hands, palms facing inwards. Move the flesh between your hands with circular movements, pressing inwards. Your hands should shift down the foot from the toes to the ankle as you massage — similar in movement to a train in motion.

This is known as palmar kneading.

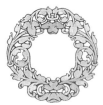

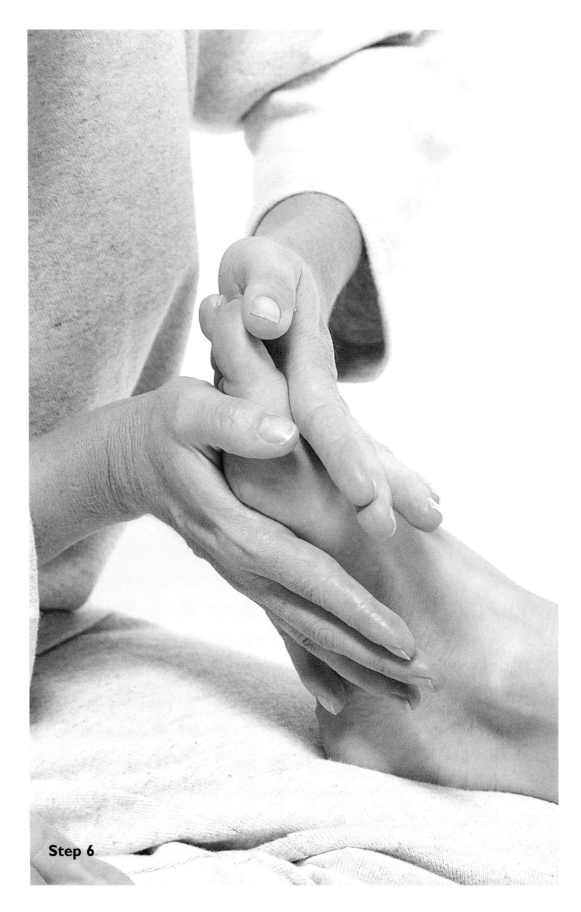

Step 6

*The feet get very cold so if they feel icy after massaging,
they may need to be covered with a folded blanket or warmed with
a hot water bottle wrapped in a towel.*

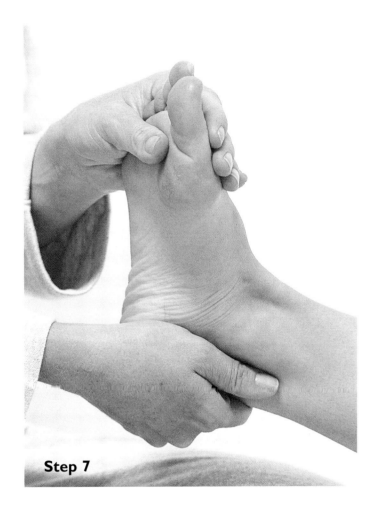

Step 7

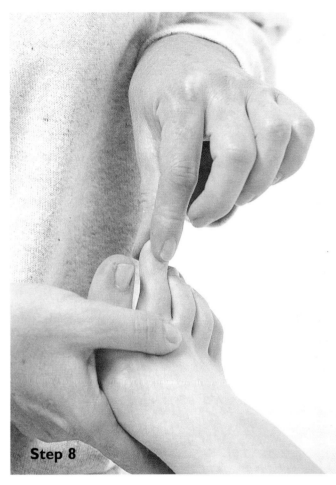

Step 8

7. Support the foot with one hand on the Achilles tendon (just above the ankle bone at the back of the leg).

Rotate the foot in a clockwise then an anticlockwise direction.

Do not force the foot if the joint is stiff; work slowly and gently.

8. Rotate each of the toes, in both directions. While rotating with one hand, hold the base of the toe with the other hand to add support.

9. Gently pull each toe.

10. Conclude the foot massage with soothing strokes, gently gliding the hands off the ends of the toes.

11. After massaging the foot, "reunite" it with the leg by gently shaking the whole leg at the ankle, or stroking the leg from thigh to feet.

12. Cover feet and squeeze.

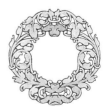

The Arm

Cover the legs and reposition yourself so that you are kneeling beside your partner's arm. Apply oil with stroking movements to the whole arm.

1. Hold the arm softly at the wrist with one hand, while effleuraging with the other. Glide from the lower arm to upper arm, around the shoulder and slide back down to the hand.

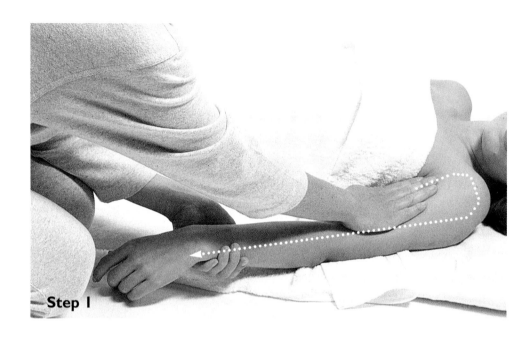

Step 1

2. Concentrate the same movements to the forearm. You may like to bend your partner's arm at the elbow and hold the wrist with one hand while the other effleurages towards the elbow and returns to the wrist.

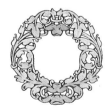

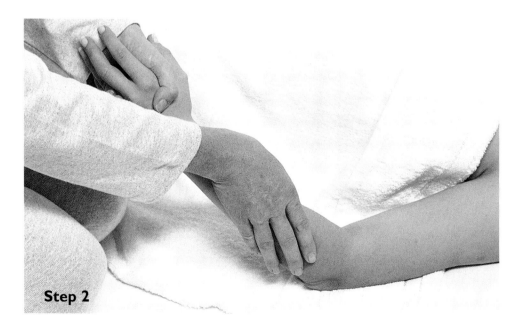

Step 2

40

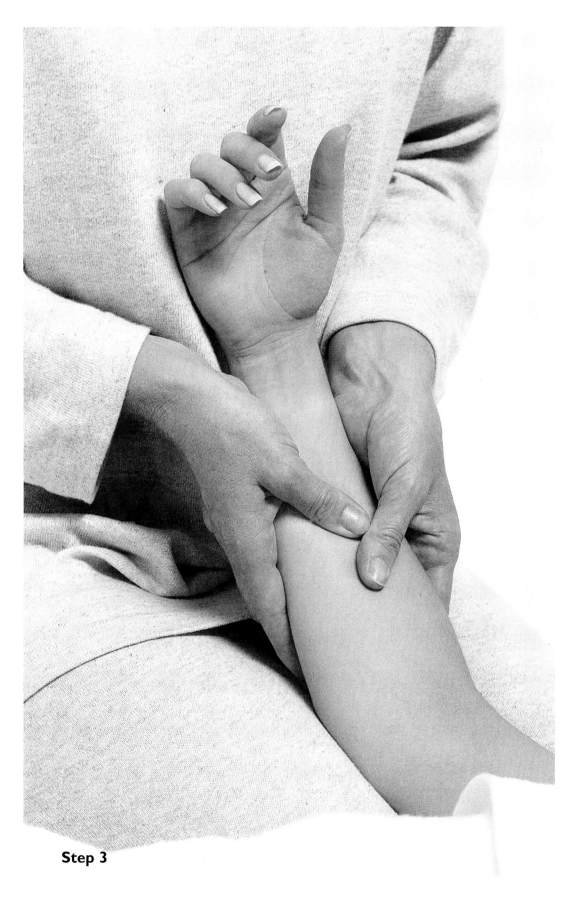

Step 3

3. Still working on the forearm, try circular friction movements to the area, on the front and then the back. Use each thumb alternately to thoroughly massage the whole area.

4. Knead the forearm by sandwiching it between your hands and squeezing in circular movements along the forearm. This is similar to the palmer kneading or "train" movements described in the foot massage (see page 38).

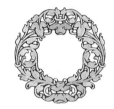

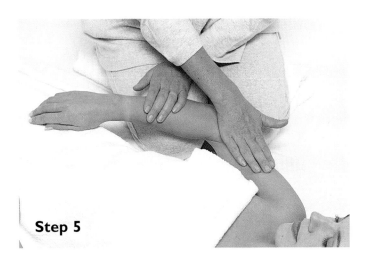

Step 5

5. Rest the forearm across your knee as shown. Now concentrate on effleurage to the upper arm.

6. Try friction movements on the upper arm's inner and outer surface along the muscles, using your thumbs and the pads of your fingers.

7. Once again, you may wish to use the train-like palmer movements as illustrated below— this time work up and down the upper arm.

8. Moving the arm off your knee, effleurage the entire arm to soothe and connect the area.

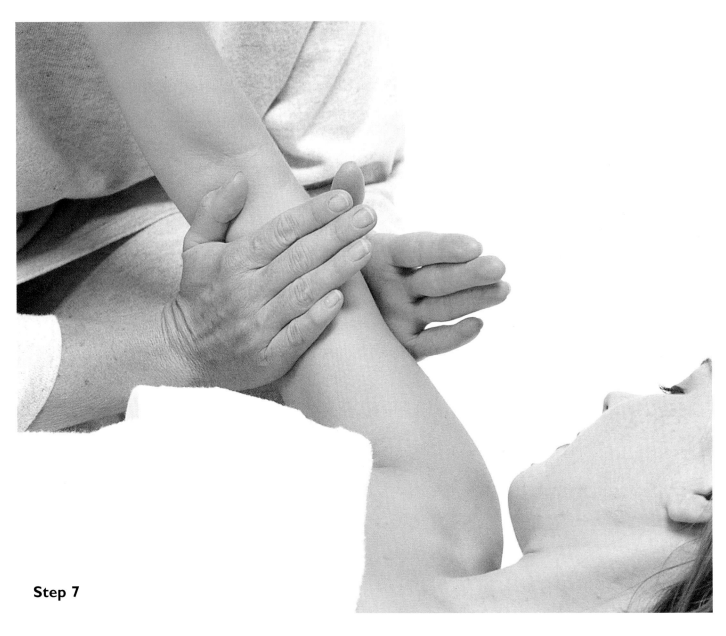

Step 7

Massage of the hands is very reassuring —
use your own intuition and create your own style.
Work on the palms, backs of hands,
and each of the fingers.

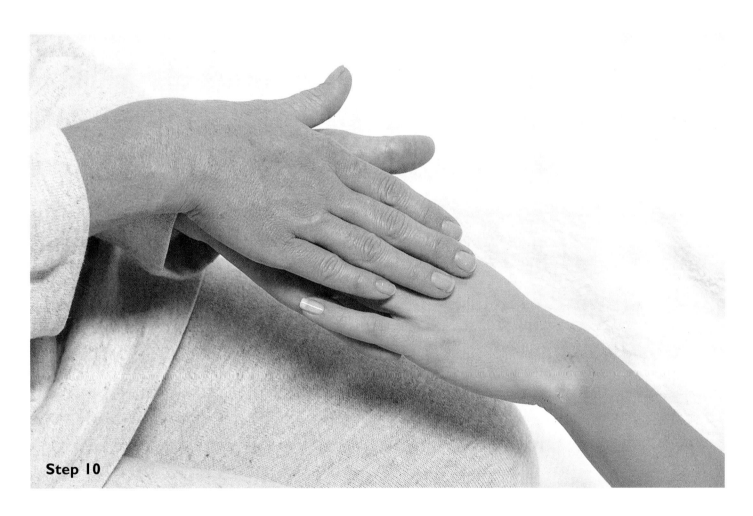

Step 10

9. Hold your partner's hand in yours and rub the palm with your thumb. Stroke the upper surface of the hand. Gently rotate the wrist. Rotate the fingers and very softly pull them away from the hands.

10. Conclude the arm massage by gently stroking from shoulders to hands. On the final stroke let your hands glide lightly off your partner's. Cover the arm with a towel and pat gently. Repeat process on the other arm.

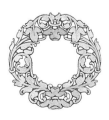

The Abdomen

If the temperature is cool, arrange towels so only the area from the rib cage to the pelvis is exposed.

1. Kneel on one side of your partner near the waist. Apply oil to the whole area with gentle, stroking movements.

2. Effleurage up the middle of the abdomen, out over the lower ribs and down towards the waist. Pull back down to the lower abdomen, and repeat the whole movement.

3. Gently knead the whole abdomen, starting at the opposite side of the body and working toward you.

4. The next movement is a deep sliding one that aims to follow the outline of the large intestine; it is very helpful for abdominal discomfort.

Using the heal of your right hand, start on the right side of your partner's abdomen and gently push up from the hip area towards the lower rib. Then glide your whole hand across the abdomen, and drag the flat of your fingers down your partner's left hand side. It is basically an upside-down U-shape, as illustrated.

5. Gently soothe the area with circular effleurage. Your hands should move alternately in wide, clockwise circles, as illustrated; one hand leaving the abdomen as the other makes contact. It is a continuous, rhythmic motion which is very calming.

6. Follow with a stretching movement. Your partner should be relaxed, and the movement is done slowly and carefully — don't pull hard. You don't need to be strong.

Lean well over your partner's body. Place one of your hands under each side of your partner's waist. Pull upwards, rising onto your knees and straightening your arms. Your partner's waist will lift off the floor, lengthening the whole abdominal region. Let go softly but allowing your hands to glide across the abdomen and meet in the middle of your partner's body. See the illustration opposite.

7. Repeat gentle kneading to the entire abdomen.

8. Finish with gentle effleurage up the middle of the abdomen, out over the lower ribs, and down to the waist.

9. Cover the area with a towel, and place both your hands on the abdomen, applying gentle pressure, before allowing the hands to lift from the area.

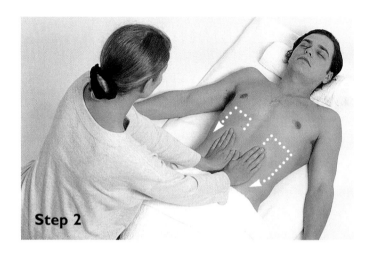

Step 2

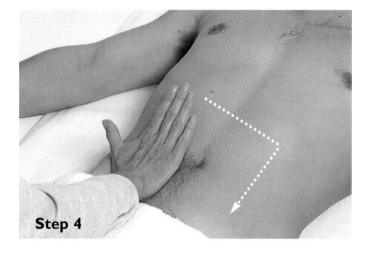

Step 4

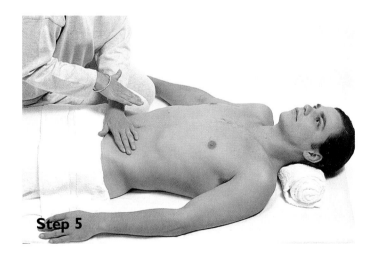

Step 5

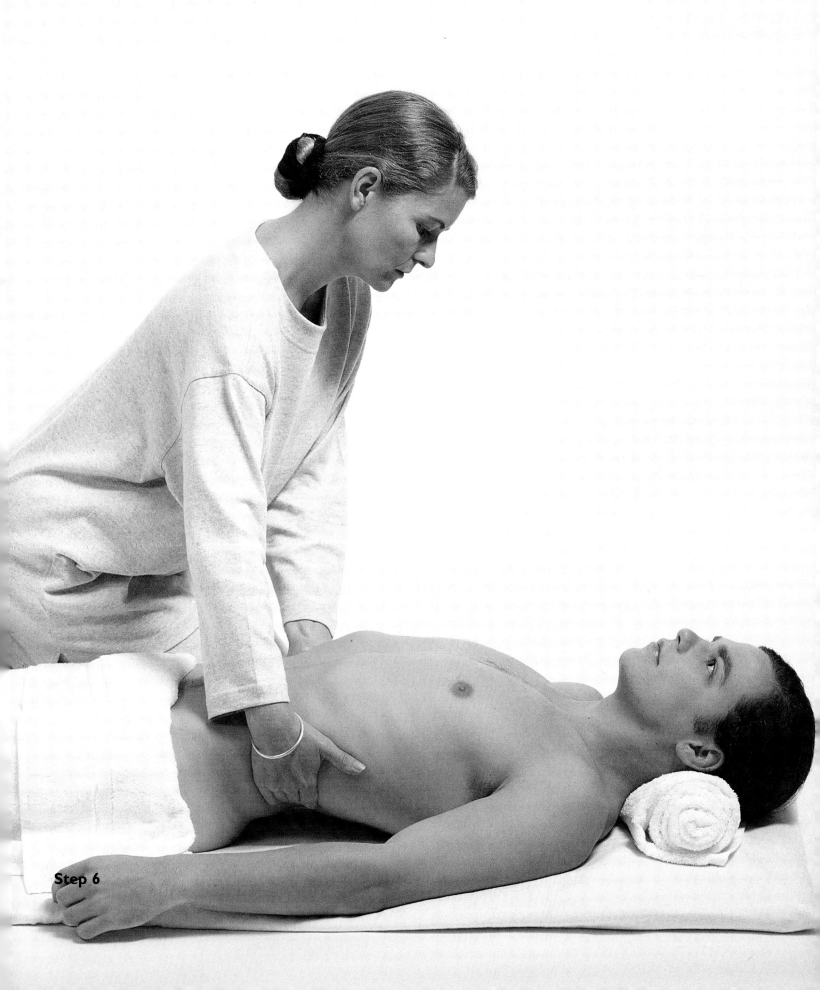

Step 6

The Chest

*A chest massage
should be included when
massaging both men
and women. If your partner
does not feel comfortable
with the chest exposed, you can
arrange towels to cover
the breasts, leaving the upper
chest area (including
the pectoral muscles) and
shoulders exposed.*

Step 1

1. Kneel at the head of your partner and apply the oil by gliding hands down the middle of chest. Separate the hands, go around the breast area and return up the sides of body.

See opposite page.

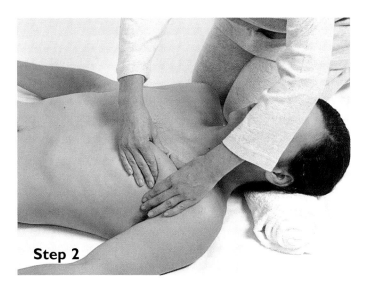

Step 2

2. Knead the upper pectoral area — the fleshy area below the collarbone. Squeeze and release the flesh using both hands alternately. Work one side fully, then the other. See above.

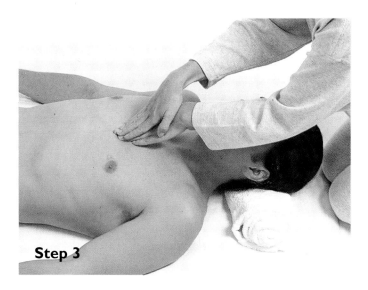

Step 3

3. Using the pads of the fingers and light pressure only, work with friction movements over the breastbone. This area can be quite tender so keep the pressure light.

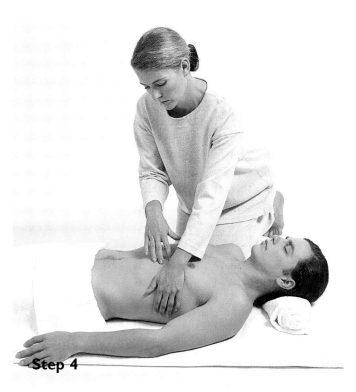

Step 4

4. Move to the side of your partner, and with the palms of your hands alternately stroke over the ribs opposite you, towards the middle of your partner's body.

Repeat on the other side.

5. Finish by repeating the movements in step 1.

6. Cover the chest and shoulders with a towel, and gently press both hands on the breastbone, then on the pectoral muscles, and gently release.

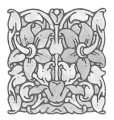

The Neck

This is a very important area, as most of us
store a lot of tension in the neck and upper shoulders.
Place a rolled towel under your partner's
head so that you can freely access the back of the neck.

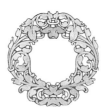

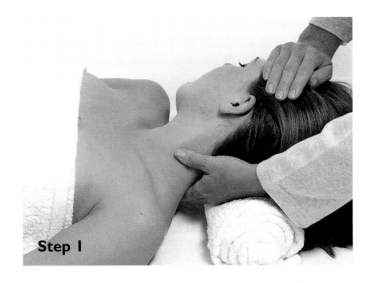

Step 1

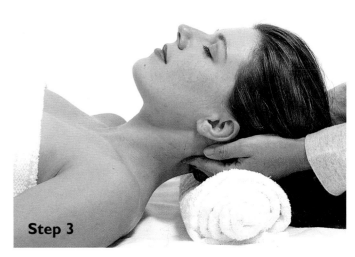

Step 3

1. Turn the head to one side and gently stroke with your thumb from the base of the skull to the collarbone.

2. While the head is in this position, knead the upper shoulder muscle. Turn the head to the other side, and repeat.

3. With the head facing straight up, place both your hands under the base of the neck, and using the pads of the fingers create circular movements up the neck to the base of the skull. The circles should be quite large.

4. Use small friction movements with the pads of the fingers along the base of the skull — work out to the ears and back. This area, where the head joins the neck, is often very tender.

5. Try a gentle neck stretch. Cup the head with both hands, making sure the head is well supported. Ask your partner to let their head be heavy, then lift the head smoothly and gently stretch it forward — see opposite. Do not use force.

6. Finish by stroking with both hands from the shoulders to the back of the scalp.

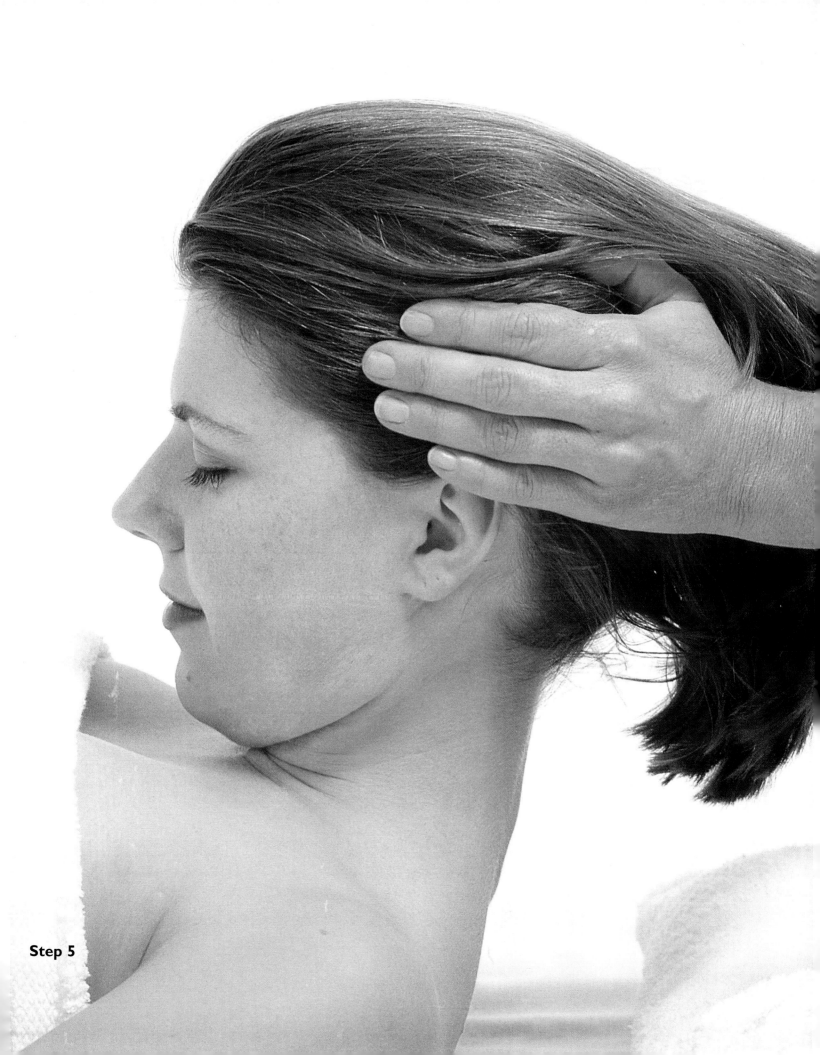

Step 5

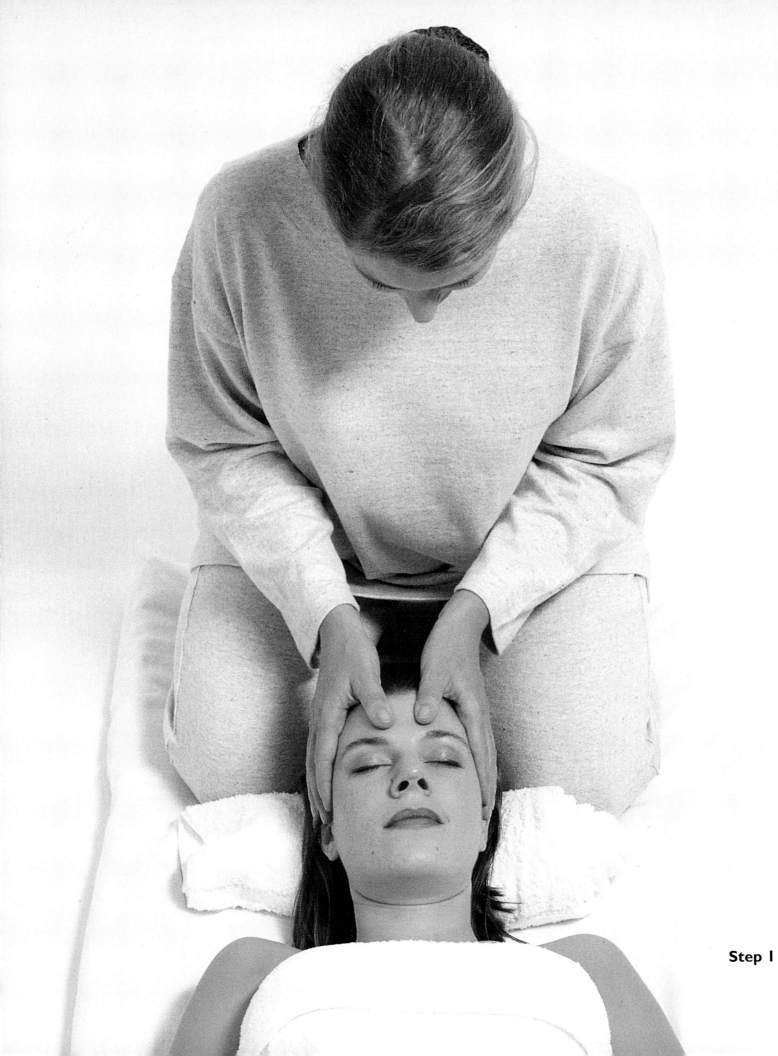

Step 1

The Face and Scalp

*It is very relaxing to conclude a massage
with the face and scalp to gently soothe away any remnants of tension
and leave your partner in a state of blissful calm.*

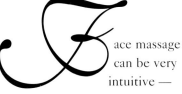ace massage can be very intuitive — don't worry too much about following a set pattern, just do what feels good at the time. You should, of course, always be gentle.

Experiment with various techniques such as pinching along the eyebrows, small frictions along the side of the nose, soft slapping to the cheeks and neck, even squeezing along the edge of the ears!

1. Sit at the head of your partner and begin with effleurage over the forehead with your thumbs.

Start with the pads of your thumbs together in the middle of the forehead and stroke out to the temple area. Stroke several times, covering the entire forehead.

2. Place your fingers under the jaw and pull along the sides of the face towards the corners of the eyes. Start with the edge of your hands touching each other and draw them away to opposite sides of the face.

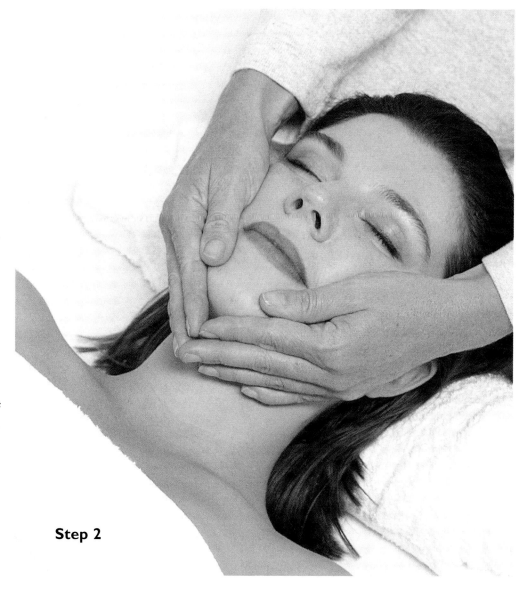

Step 2

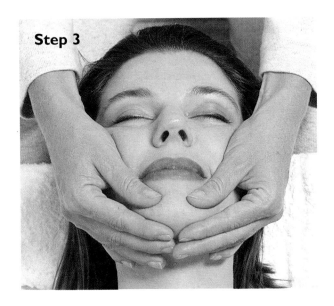

Step 3

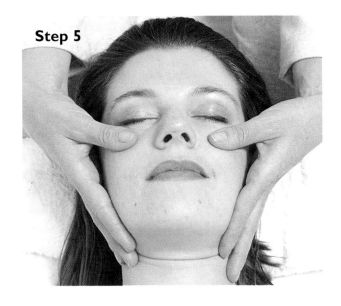

Step 5

3. Knead the chin area by gently squeezing and releasing along the jaw line. Use your thumb and fingers, and work from the middle of the chin out to the ears.

4. Using gentle friction movements with the pads of your fingers, massage around and over the mouth and cheek area.

5. Stroke with both thumbs over the arch of the cheekbone, from inside to out.

6. Massage the temple area with the pads of your thumbs, using small stationary circles.

7. Stroke over the eyebrows with your thumbs.

8. Create frictions with the pads of your fingers over the forehead and the scalp.

9. Now apply thumb pressure to the forehead and scalp. Start at the middle of the forehead with both your thumbs together and work back into the scalp as far as possible. Separate thumbs slightly and work back again. Repeat until the whole area has been worked.

10. Massage the entire scalp in a "shampooing" motion.

11. Gently stroke the forehead with the heels of your thumbs and the side of the face with your fingers.

12. Use long soft strokes from the neck to the jawline.

13. Rub your hands together until they are very warm, and hold them on your partner's face. They should completely cover the face but only just touch. Hold for a minute, allowing your partner to drink in the warmth.

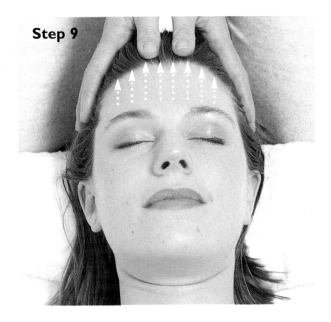

Step 9

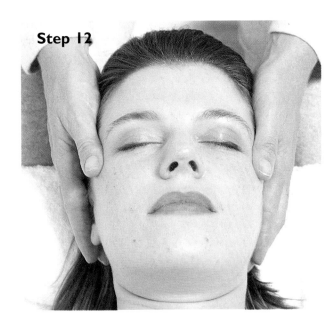

Step 12

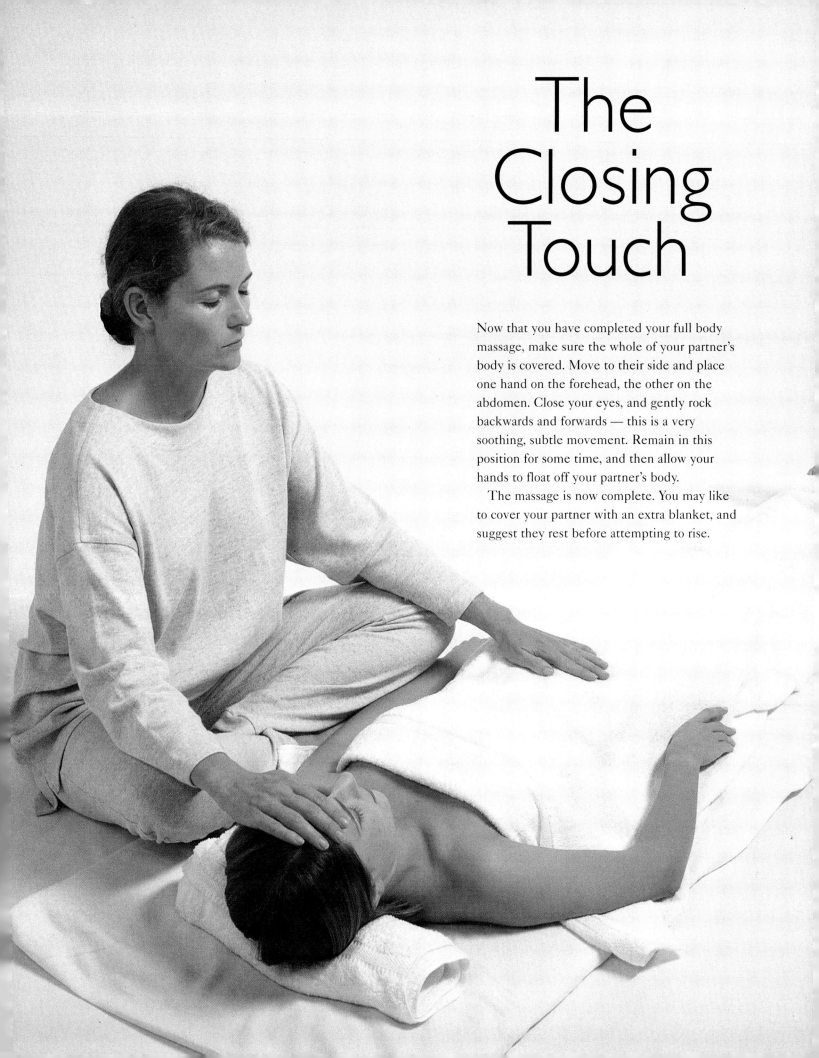

The Closing Touch

Now that you have completed your full body massage, make sure the whole of your partner's body is covered. Move to their side and place one hand on the forehead, the other on the abdomen. Close your eyes, and gently rock backwards and forwards — this is a very soothing, subtle movement. Remain in this position for some time, and then allow your hands to float off your partner's body.

The massage is now complete. You may like to cover your partner with an extra blanket, and suggest they rest before attempting to rise.

A seated massage can be given anytime, anywhere to help soothe tight and tense muscles. It is great for combating fatigue and daily stress.

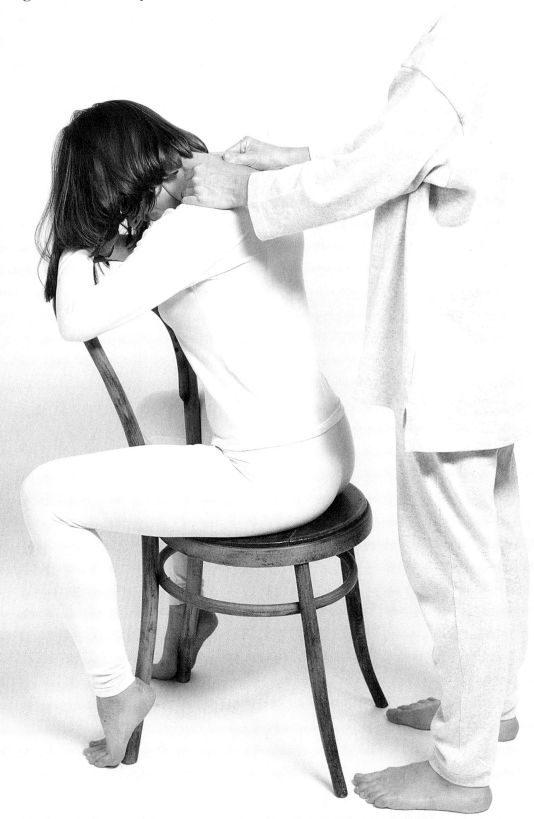

Step 1

A Quick, Do-Anywhere Massage

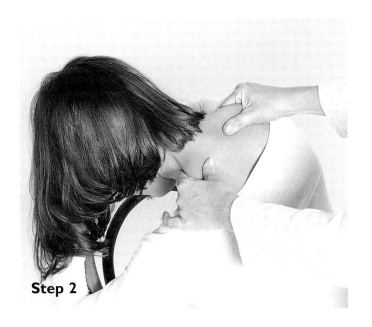

Step 2

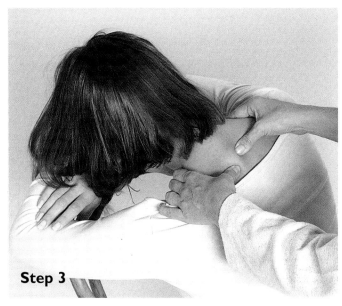

Step 3

This massage can be performed at work, at home, at a friend's house, and the receiver may remain fully clothed. The massage may take only five to ten minutes in time, but will give hours of relief.

It is best to have your partner sit astride a chair, with arms folded and head resting on the arms. A cushion or pillow can add extra comfort.

1. Start at the shoulders using kneading movements. Squeeze and release with both hands at the same time. Work the whole shoulder area and then continue down the upper arms.

2. Using small, deep friction movements with your thumbs, work the shoulder area and base of the neck.

3. Place one thumb on each side of the base of the neck, and apply firm pressure — hold the thumbs still and use your body weight for strength. Move your thumbs down the spine a little then reapply pressure. Continue with thumb pressures down each side of the spine till you are parallel with the end of the shoulder blade.

4. With the same movement, work along the inside edge of the shoulder blade, moving upwards toward the top of the shoulder.

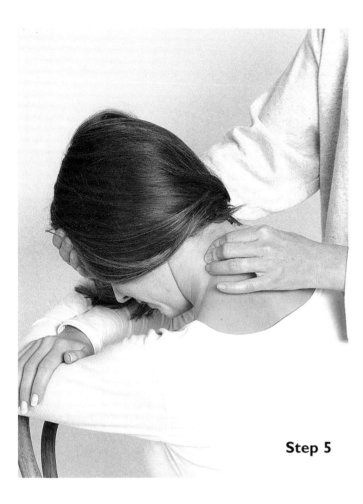

Step 5

5. Place the palm of one hand on your partner's forehead for support, and knead the base of the neck with the other hand.

6. Continue kneading up the neck to the base of the skull.

7. Using the pads of your fingers, create circular friction movements over the whole scalp area.

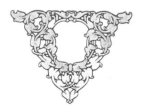

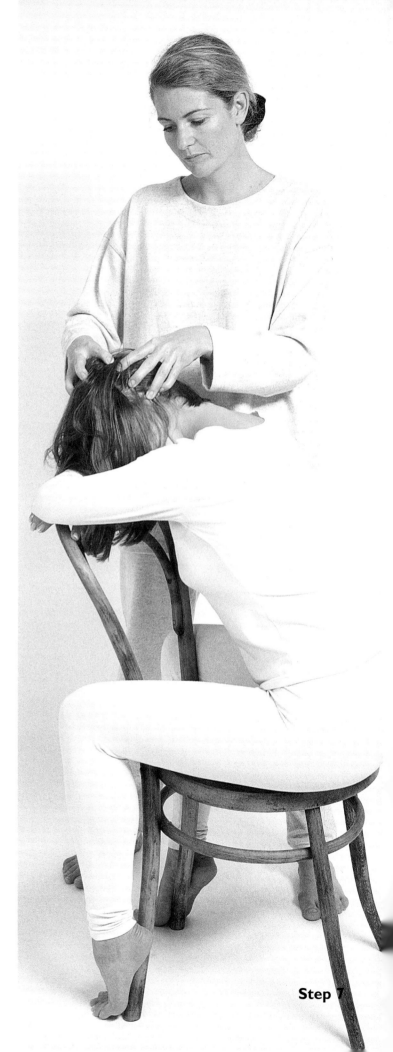

Step 7

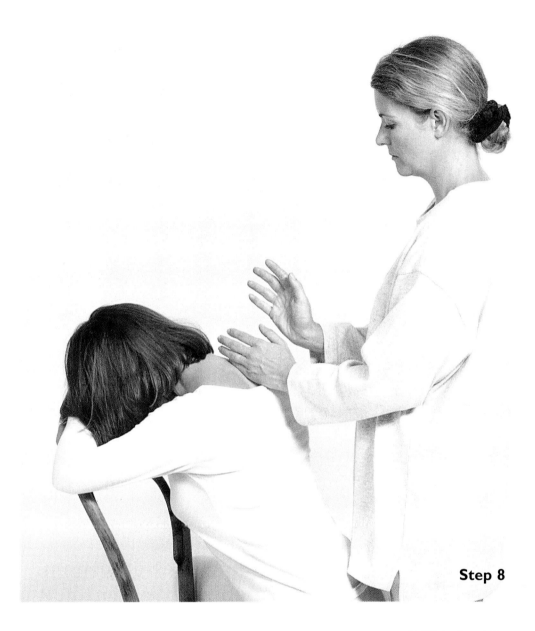

8. Now return to the shoulders and apply gentle flicking movements to the whole of the upper back.

Your hands should be relaxed, with palms facing one another and the wrists should be soft.

Create a light, fast, bouncy movement using the little finger edge of the hands. Be careful to avoid bony areas.

This movement will help to invigorate your partner.

Step 8

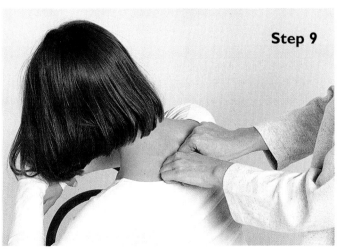

Step 9

9. With closed fists, gently press in with knuckles each side of spine from the base of the neck to below the scapula.

10. Soothe the area with more kneading to the shoulders and down the arms.

11. Conclude the massage with light stroking over the whole area.

Your friend will be ready to face the world with reduced stress and far more energy.

Self Massage

Self massage can help to soothe away the tensions of the day,
and is very useful if there is no massage partner on hand.
Before you begin, close your eyes and breathe deeply for a few minutes.

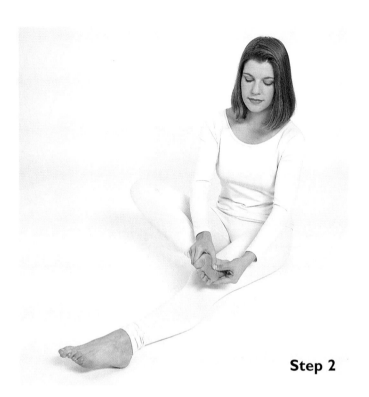

Step 2

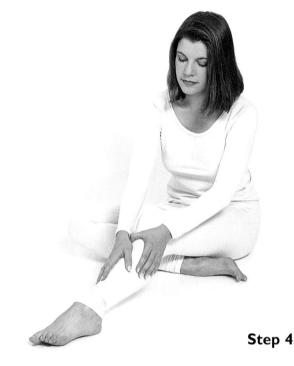

Step 4

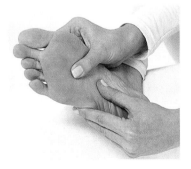

Feet and legs

1. Sit on the floor with one leg comfortably extended and bend the other leg so you can grasp the foot. Stroke the sole of the foot with one hand.

2. Apply deeper thumb pressures using both thumbs, as illustrated. Use small, penetrating circles, covering the entire sole.

3. Firmly squeeze over the whole of your foot using both hands.

4. With your knee bent, reach out with both hands to the foot. In one long, smooth movement, stroke up the front of the leg over the shin, knee, and thigh.

5. Repeat but this time stroke up the back of the leg.

6. Next concentrate on the calf muscle, effleuraging deeply from foot to knee.

7. Move up to the thigh and repeat the deep effleurage movement, pulling from knee to groin.

8. Give the thigh area a good knead. Work the outside of the muscle mass using thumb and fingers, alternately squeezing and releasing, as illustrated opposite. This movement adds tone to the thigh muscle.

9. Repeat the whole process to your other leg.

*When you are
massaging yourself,
try to clear your
mind and focus on
the sensation alone.
It is important
to be comfortable,
and to keep
all your muscles
relaxed.*

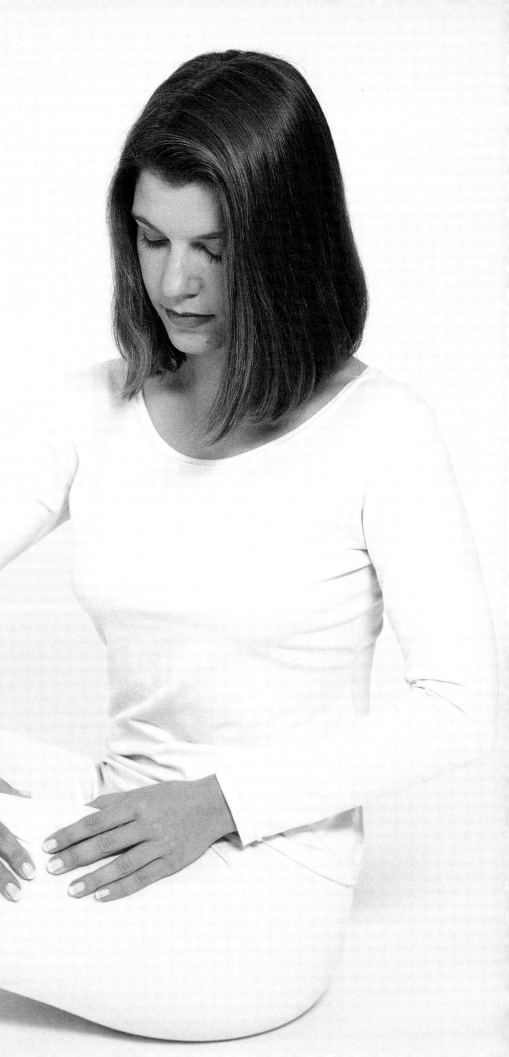

For massaging the abdomen and chest, you may wish to lie on your back with a pillow or rolled towel under your knees and your head.

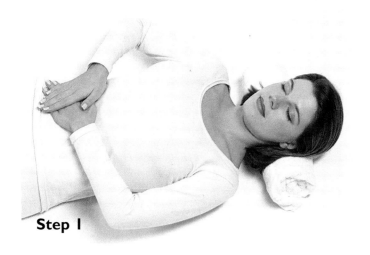

Step 1

Abdomen and chest

1. With one hand on top of the other, create clockwise circular movements over the abdomen.

2. Gently pinch the whole of the abdominal area, including the waist, using thumb and index fingers.

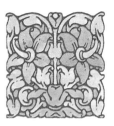

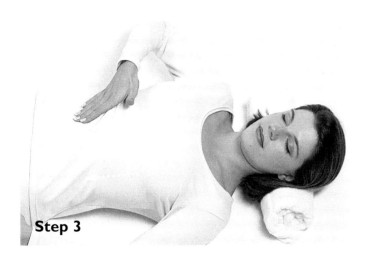

Step 3

3. Next give attention to your whole large intestine (colon) which runs in the shape of an inverted "U" up the right side of the abdomen, across, and down the left side. Massaging this area is invaluable in times of abdominal discomfort.

With the fingers of the right hand pull up from the groin area to the ribcage, push across abdomen to left side, and then stroke down with the heel of left hand from ribs to groin area.

This movement should be done quite deeply and firmly, to stimulate the internal organs.

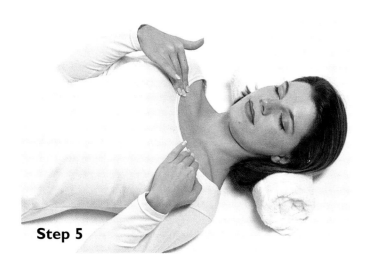

Step 5

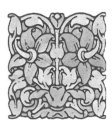

4. Moving up to the chest, massage the breastbone gently with the fingertips of both hands.

5. Now apply small, circular frictions with fingertips around the chest muscles and under the collarbone on both sides of body.

For the upper body, you may wish to remain lying down or sit upright. It is very soothing to keep the eyes closed.

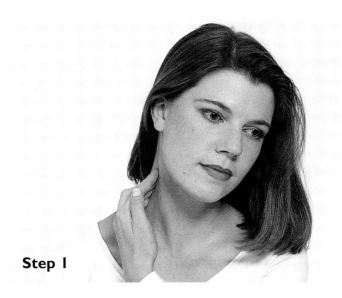

Step 1

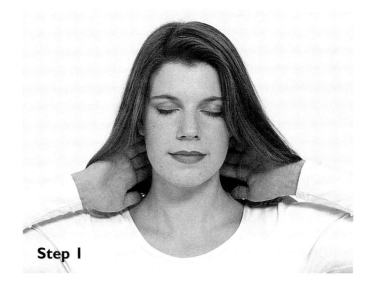

Step 1

Neck, shoulders, and arms

1. With palm and fingers, stroke from the base of your scalp to the collarbone. This will gently relax the neck muscles. Work both sides.

2. Bringing one hand across your body to your other shoulder, knead the area by sqeezing and releasing.

3. Continue this movement all the way down the arm to the wrist, and then back up again.

4. Now, work your shoulder area more deeply, with fingertip frictions.

5. Repeat steps 2 to 4 to other side of your body, using the other hand.

Scalp

1. Moving to the base of your skull, start just behind the ears and work aound the ridge to the middle of your neck, using small deep finger frictions. You are likely to find many tender spots in this area. If you find one, work gradually to soothe away the tension.

2. Follow this movement with a relaxing massage to the whole scalp, using all your fingers in small circular movements. Feel the skin move under your fingertips.

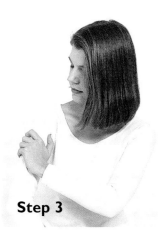

Step 3

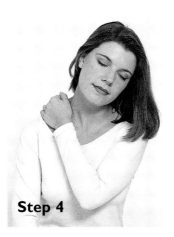

Step 4

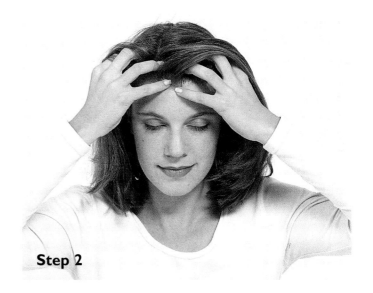

Step 2

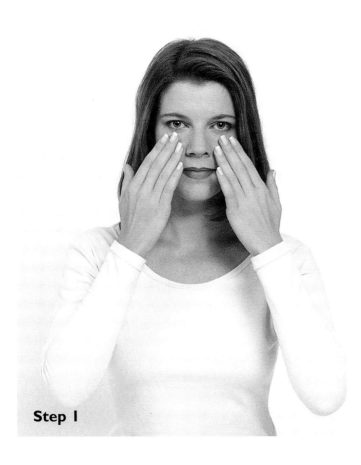

Step I

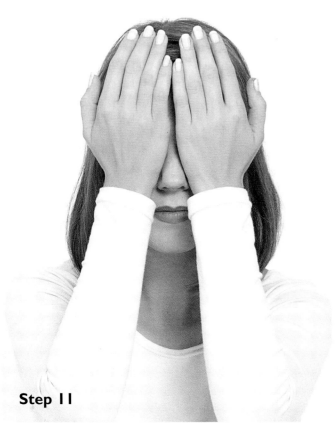

Step II

Very gently caress your whole face to complete your massage.

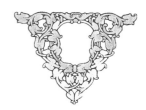

1. Stroke over the cheek area with your fingertips.

2. Smooth the nose area and over your lips with your fingertips.

3. Stroke along your jawline from chin out to your ears.

4. Knead the chin area by gently squeezing and releasing along the jawline. Use your thumbs and fingers and work from the chin out to the ears.

5. Squeeze along the edge of your ears.

6. Very gently "slap" your face, your cheeks, and neck.

7. With small circular movements, massage the mouth and cheek area.

8. Use the same movements to massage along the sides of your nose.

9. Very carefully massage around the eyes with the pads of fingers, not forgetting to stroke your eyelids.

10. Stroke over your eyebrows with your fingers.

11. Rub your hands together until they are warm, and then place palms or fingers over your eyes, applying a gentle pressure. Stay like this for a minute or so. Feel the penetrating warmth. It is surprising how comforting and relaxing this simple movement is. You can use it during the day to relieve tired eyes.

12. Using your index or middle fingers, press each side of the eyesocket at the top of your nose, as illustrated. Be careful of long fingernails. Hold for several seconds.

13. Now massage the whole of your forehead and temple area using the pads of fingers in small circular movements.

14. Finish by gently stroking your entire face, and running fingers softly down your throat.

15. Your self massage is now complete. Allow yourself some time to relax before slowly rising.

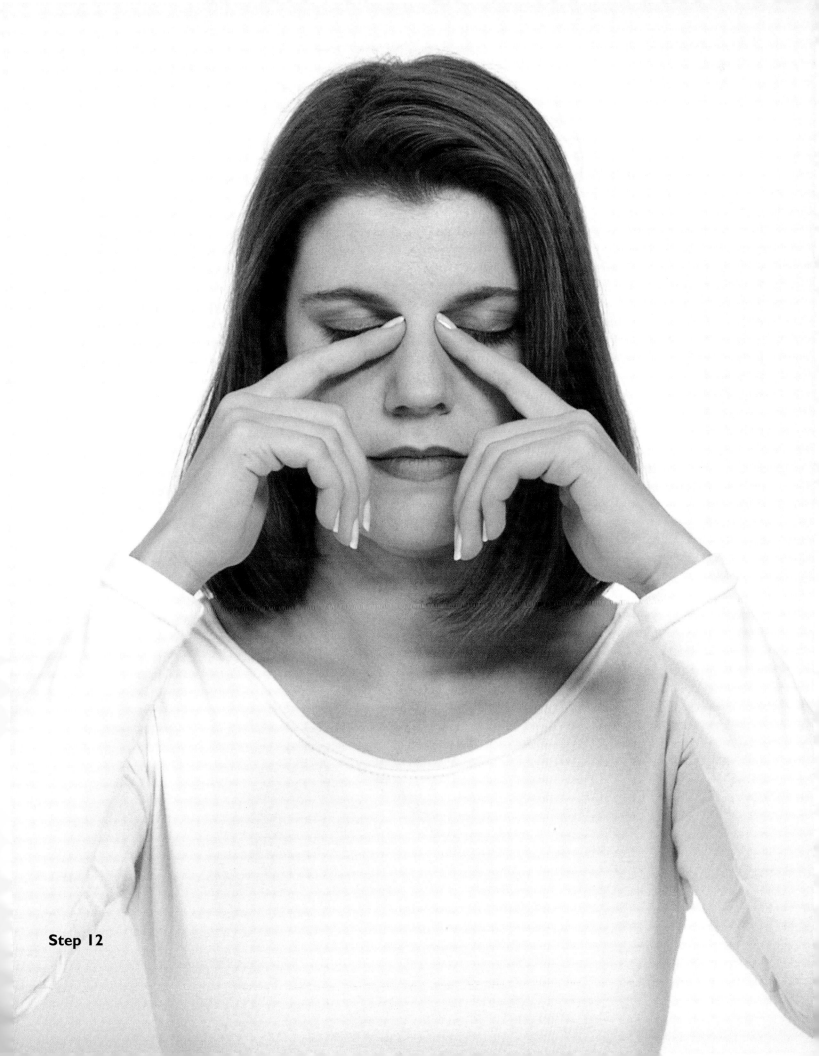

Step 12

Acknowledgments

*The expert guidance of Allan Hudson of Naturecare College
is greatly appreciated by the publishers, as is the contribution of Karen Bailey.*

*The publishers are also very grateful to Niki Barnes
for her patience and assistance in demonstrating massage techniques in the photographs.*

Thanks too to Michael Tilgals for his assistance.

Published by Lansdowne Publishing Pty Ltd
Level 5, 70 George Street, Sydney, NSW 2000, Australia
Chief Executive Publisher: Jane Curry
Publishing Manager: Deborah Nixon
Production Manager: Sally Stokes
Project Co-ordinator: Kirsten Tilgals
Project Assistant: Amalia Matheson
Project consultant: Karen Bailey
Designer: Michelle Wiener
Photographer: André Martin
Stylist: Mary-Anne Danaher

First published in 1996
© Copyright: Lansdowne Publishing Pty Ltd

Set in Caslon 540 Roman on Quark Xpress
Printed in Singapore by Tien Wah Press (Pte) Ltd

National Library of Australia Cataloguing-in-Publication Data
The relaxing art of massage.
ISBN 1 86302 465 4.
1. Massage.
615.822